A Gaia Busy Person's Guide

Reflexology

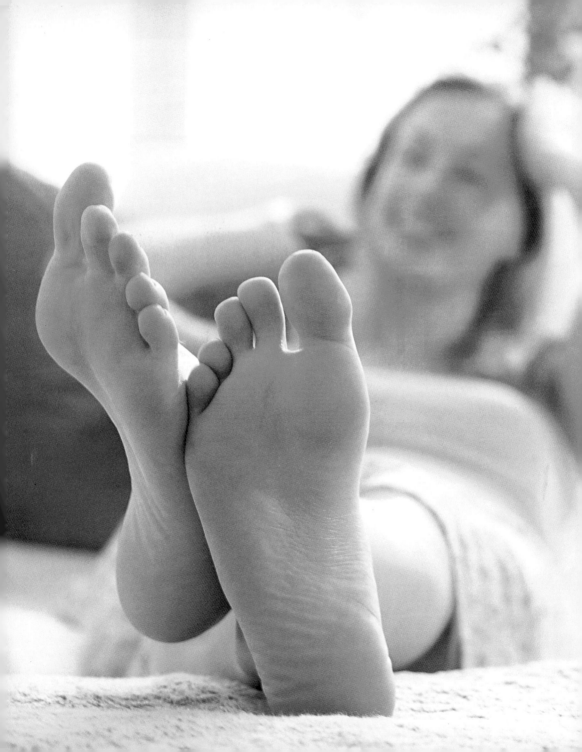

A Gaia **Busy Person's** Guide

Reflexology

Simple routines for home, work, & travel

Ann Gillanders

Gaia Books

A Gaia Original

Books from Gaia celebrate the vision of Gaia, the self-sustaining living Earth, and seek to help its readers live in greater personal and planetary harmony.

Editor Susanna Abbott
Designer Phil Gamble
Photography Dominic Blackmore, Gus Filgate, Mark Preston
Production Lyn Kirby
Editorial direction Jo Godfrey Wood
Direction Patrick Nugent

® This is a Registered Trade Mark of Gaia Books an imprint of Octopus Publishing Group.
2–4 Heron Quays, London E14,4JP

First published in the United Kingdom in 2002 by Gaia Books Ltd.

ISBN-13 9 781856 752510
ISBN 1-85675-251-8

A catalogue record of this book is available from the British Library.

Printed and bound in China

10 9 8 7 6 5 4 3 2 1

Contents

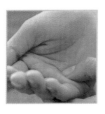 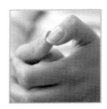 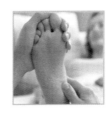 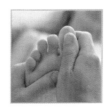

Using this book

This book offers reflexology techniques to fit around your busy working day, from the moment you wake up in the morning until you close your eyes at night, supported by health advice and simple natural therapies. It is both a quick reference manual and a lifestyle guide: you can dip into it during the day if you need to relieve a specific condition or you can use it to guide you systematically through the day for an all-round healthy life.

Because it is not normally practical to treat the feet until you are relaxing at home, the author has selected simple hand treatments that are ideal for self-help during the day. Foot reflexology is reserved

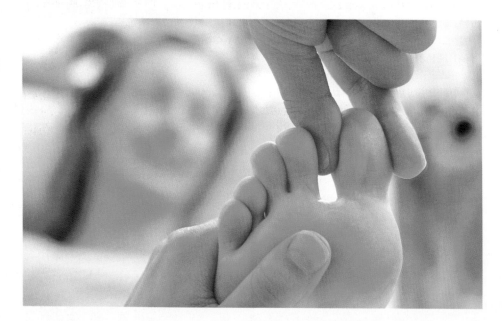

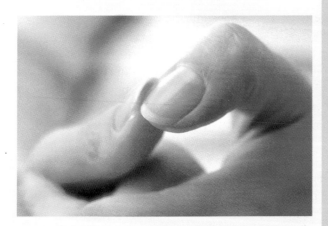

for evenings and weekends, when you have the time to relax properly and share a treatment with a partner, as you cannot effectively treat your own feet.

Chapter One explains how reflexology works and the general techniques you will need to treat yourself or a loved one. It is important to read this chapter before attempting any of the treatments in the rest of the book. Chapter Two shows you how to start your day and includes self-help hand treatments. Chapter Three will help you make any journey as comfortable and as safe as possible, has self-help treatments as well as a complete hand treatment. Chapter Four guides you through your day in the office, while the complete foot treatment in Chapter Five will let you banish the most stressful of days. Chapter Six is a reference section to treat and prevent specific conditions, concentrating on foot reflexology.

CAUTION
This book is not intended to replace medical care under the direct supervision of a qualified doctor. Before embarking on any changes in your health regime, consult your doctor.

Equally, whilst reflexology is an extremely safe therapy, you must seek professional advice if you are in any doubt about any medical condition, particularly if you or the person to be treated suffers from diabetes, thrombosis, or phlebitis, or are undergoing conventional treatments for cancer. Do not treat people in the acute stage of any infectious disease and always seek advice from a professional reflexologist before treating women during the first 14 weeks of pregnancy, particularly if they have a history of miscarriage. Any application of the ideas and information contained in this book is at the reader's sole discretion and risk.

Introduction

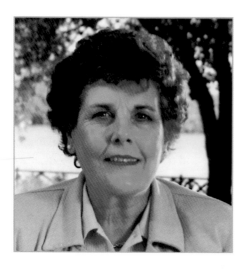

Reflexology is one of the most powerful natural therapies for counteracting the stress and tensions of modern life. Easy to use and deeply relaxing, it works to restore your body's power to heal itself.

UNDERSTANDING STRESS
Our hectic modern lifestyles are highly stimulating, but we are often unable, or we forget, to relax properly: we have become used to existing in a perpetual state of nervous tension and think we need high levels of stress in our daily lives to function "normally".

Nonetheless, we tend to think of stress as a very negative influence in our lives.

How often do we hear ourselves or our friends saying, "I can't come out—I had a really tiring, stressful day at work", "I feel stressed", "I can't cope with travelling in rush hour traffic—it's too stressful", or "I just need some time to myself to unwind"? In moderation stress is actually a positive influence in our lives and a great motivator. Generally, daily pressures keep us moving and growing: they ensure we arrive at work on time or successfully organize a dinner party for a group of friends.

However, it is also true that too much stress can disturb the body's normal functioning, typically affecting sleeping patterns, and the digestive and immune systems, and causing anxiety or depression.

OVERREACTION
Unfortunately, because we are so busy, many of us tend to overreact to everyday pressures and respond very negatively to only modestly stressful situations. Constant overreaction, either physically or emotionally, to daily frustrations makes us highly strung and unnecessarily aggressive: road rage in commuter traffic, tears over a computer failure, or shouting at waiting staff in

restaurants over bad service are classic examples. It is not only exhausting to feel permanently on edge, but also bad for our long-term health. This is because the body reacts instinctively to high levels of stress and channels resources away from less essential functions to the parts of the body that are most needed to fight in or flee from the situation. This in turn weakens the immune system and leaves us vulnerable to illness— someone who is tired out and stressed is more likely to get flu than someone who is relaxed and happy. Generally, if a person is frequently ill or suffers from any stress-related ailments, such as migraine, asthma, skin disorders, high blood pressure, or irritable bowel syndrome, steps should be taken to treat the source of the condition and not just the immediate physical symptoms.

BEAT STRESS WITH REFLEXOLOGY

The ancient practice of reflexology is ideal for treating and preventing stress-related problems, for not only does it treat the immediate physical condition but it also helps the patient relax, thereby treating the root cause, stress. In this way, reflexology treats the whole person and not just the local symptom.

Reflexology is a completely safe and non-invasive therapy that works by applying pressure to specific reflex points on the feet and hands. Each reflex point corresponds to a part of the body (see pp.26–33). Working these reflex points stimulates the nerve endings and blood circulation as well as alleviating stress and tension held in the body.

Although a foot treatment is the most effective form of reflexology (see p.16), there are many hand exercises you can do on yourself during the day to help you relax and relieve problems such as migraine, indigestion, and back pain.

Stop for a moment and consider at which point during the day you begin to feel drained and lose your concentration. If you need a boost at the beginning of your day, try a quick five-minute routine in the morning to energize yourself, concentrating on the spinal area on your hands (see pp.38–9). Contacting the spine reflex stimulates all the parts of the body to work in harmony.

Many people have a dip in energy after lunch. If you always feel tired in the afternoon, your digestive system may be the problem—perhaps you ate a hurried lunch at your desk. Work the liver, stomach, and intestinal reflexes for five to ten minutes to bring relief. Allowing yourself the luxury of a treatment is also great for morale, and you will find you can face the rest of the day with a wholly positive attitude.

If you have had a particularly tough day at work ask your partner or a friend to give you a complete foot reflexology treatment at home (see pp.86–101). All you need is a comfortable chair or sofa and a couple of cushions to elevate the feet. Not only will you experience the full benefits of reflexology but you will also draw great comfort from the healing power of touch. If you are very busy and have to go out in the evenings, try setting aside time at the weekend and take it in turns to treat each other.

REASSESS YOUR LIFESTYLE
Because reflexology is a holistic therapy, treating the entire person and not just any one symptom, it is also important that you consider your general lifestyle when overcoming a condition. For example, if you suffer from stress-related migraine, ask yourself what simple steps you can take to reduce unnecessary stress in your life. This might be a combination of simple changes, for example, ironing your shirt or making

your lunch the night before so you have less to do in the morning, or you may need to consider making more fundamental changes in your life, such as finding another job or moving house.

LEARN TO RELAX
You must also learn how to relax properly, as this is the key to finding balance in a busy lifestyle. If you are relaxed you can put problems into perspective, release pent-up frustrations, and safeguard your health. Make sure that you give yourself time every day to unwind. Meditation, yoga, and tai chi are all excellent ways to help you leave behind the worries of your day. If you prefer to sit quietly on your own at home, try evaporating a couple of drops of rose, neroli, ylang ylang, or lavender essential oils in an aromatherapy burner whilst listening to your favourite soothing music or reading a novel.

WORK IT OUT
It is vital to take some regular exercise to use up all the extra energy that your body produces when under stress. It also makes you feel more energetic during the day and helps you sleep

soundly at night. Jogging, fast walking, a session at the local gym, or swimming, are great stress relievers, as are aerobics, martial arts, dancing, or simply hitting a ball against a wall. If on some days you don't fancy exercise, simply roar out your frustration under your duvet!

EAT WELL

A good diet that is as natural as possible is key to good health (see also pp.102–3). Eat plenty of fresh fruit and vegetables every day, raw as often as possible, as well as pulses, grains, wholemeal bread, and rice. You should also drink at least 2 litres (3½ pints) of pure, filtered water each day. Try to drink most of this amount in the morning and only a little in the early evening to avoid making your kidneys work hard late at night and then having to wake up and go to the bathroom.

Avoid deep-fried foods and all processed foods, which are often low in nutrients and contain high levels of salt, saturated fats, and artificial flavourings and preservatives. These as well as too much refined sugar can help weaken the immune system. Also, think about taking a mineral and vitamin supplement, as the food we eat loses

some of its nutritional value if it is treated with chemical pesticides and fertilizers or if it has been harvested prematurely for transportation from overseas. Try to eat locally grown, organic food whenever you can.

SLEEP IT OFF

Getting regular quality sleep makes the world of difference. Some people need more or less than others, but eight hours is usually enough. If you have problems sleeping (see also pp.106–7) make sure you are properly relaxed before you climb into bed. A relaxing aromatherapy bath or massage (see p.101) will often help.

REFLEXOLOGY AND OTHER THERAPIES

Reflexology can be used in combination with most other practical therapies, such as aromatherapy, massage, reiki, shiatsu, acupuncture, acupressure, or yoga. It is quite safe to have reflexology when you are receiving homeopathy or herbalism, although you should always consult your practitioner first.

AROMATHERAPY

Essential oils are extremely versatile and can be used to heal the body and mind in baths, inhalations, massage, hot and cold compresses, and beauty products, as well as to clean and freshen your home. Although there are a few exceptions, such as lavender and tea tree oil, you should always dilute essential oils before applying them to the skin. You must follow the instructions accompanying each oil, as some are toxic and can make you feel nauseous if used in excess.

In terms of reflexology, you should never use oils when working the foot or hand as it prevents proper contact with the reflexes and makes the skin slippery. Instead, diffuse a few drops of an essential oil in an aromatherapy burner during a treatment. For example, bergamot or grapefruit oil will help revive flagging spirits and restore your energy levels, while lavender or ylang ylang promote relaxation and help you unwind.

MASSAGE

Massage works particularly well in combination with reflexology. After a foot reflexology session, ask the giver to massage the parts of your body that were particularly painful or tense on the corresponding areas of your feet.

Often it is the shoulders, back, and neck that need attention (see p.101). Massage in general is an excellent stress-buster and will relieve any tension you hold in the shoulders and neck as well as general aches, pains, and stiffness. Work the body with the flat of your hand. Try adding a few drops of aromatherapy oils in your carrier oil to enhance the massage. Oil of cloves is particularly useful for stiffness and inflammation in and around the spinal area, and lavender oil is an all-round anti-inflammatory oil that will promote good sleep. Reflexology followed by an aromatherapy massage can be particularly helpful if you suffer from insomnia (see also pp.106–7).

MEDITATION

If you find it hard to unwind and calm your mind, try meditation (see p.85). Choose a quiet, warm room and burn a few drops of your favourite incense or essential oils to help you. You may find it useful to create a small altar to focus on. Place simple objects on it, such as a lighted candle or some fresh flowers. Start by sitting for ten to 15 minutes and gradually build up until you can sit for 30 minutes. Spending a few minutes in stillness every day will clear your mind, release tension held in your body, and recharge your batteries.

A HEALTHY AND HAPPY LIFESTYLE

So, if you are tired out by the pace of life and suffer from any kind of stress-related condition, try reflexology to restore your sense of well-being. You will find that, in combination with a good diet, regular exercise, and quality sleep, reflexology will make a permanent change in your life: you will feel more energetic, more positive, and generally happier and healthier. All it takes is a few minutes every day and a desire to take control of your life.

This book guides you through the day, with each chapter showing you how to make simple yet effective changes to your daily routine. This includes everything from a quick five-minute energizing reflexology treatment when you wake up to advice on what to eat, how to survive long journeys, and how to treat problems, such as back pain, panic attacks, eye strain, and indigestion. However, before you discover how to survive life in the fast lane, make sure you familiarize yourself with the basic reflexology know-how in Chapter One.

ANN GILLANDERS

Introducing reflexology

There are thousands of pinhead-sized reflex points on the feet and hands, each relating to different organs, functions, and parts of the body. In reflexology, pressure is applied to these points to stimulate the nervous system and corresponding part of the body.

By stimulating the reflexes on the top, bottom, and inside and outside edges of the feet and hands, reflexology helps the body expel toxins, release tension, and restore its natural state of balance.

If a part of your body is inflamed, congested, or holds tension, the corresponding reflexes react sensitively to pressure. In this way your feet and hands can tell an accurate story about your health (see maps, pp.26-33).

Sensitivity can also be an early warning of more serious illness. If the imbalance is treated promptly with reflexology, it is often corrected and the illness prevented altogether. Equally, reflexology can detect past injuries to the body, as any scar tissue remaining in the body creates sensitivity in the reflexes.

Reflexology is centuries old. Inscriptions dating from 2330BC on the Tomb of the Physicians in Ankomohor, Egypt, are the earliest records of it in use. One scene shows people receiving treatment on the hands and feet. Chinese acupuncturists also used reflexology in the fourth century AD to complement their work. They applied direct pressure to the feet when the needles were in place to help release energy and induce healing.

Eunice Ingham, an American physiotherapist, introduced the West to modern reflexology in the 1930s. She learned about and refined reflexology from ancient foot maps. Today, reflexology is taught all over the world and is one of the most popular forms of complementary medicine.

How reflexology works

Although scientific research has been unable to prove how reflexology, acupuncture, or similar therapies work, cellular memory—the way the brain stores and retrieves information—offers a helpful and credible explanation. Because the brain records all of our experiences, it also remembers things that have obviously changed or we think we have forgotten.

For this reason, people who lose a limb often experience phantom pain where the limb once was, while others under hypnosis can sometimes recall traumatic, yet apparently forgotten, events in the past. This suggests that physical illness can also leave its memory of inflammation, tension, and congestion in the brain cells.

In reflexology the congested part of the body manifests itself as sensitive hand and foot reflex points. When these are stimulated, the nervous system sends a new, correct message to the brain. With frequent treatment the cell memory changes and the function of the body is restored. The reflex points that were previously very sensitive also become non-reactive.

Reflexology is a holistic therapy, treating the cause of the entire body's imbalance and not just suppressing the local pain with drugs or removing the ailing part of the body.

HANDS OR FEET?

Reflexology is most effective when given to the feet, as the feet are much more sensitive than the hands—try dipping your hands into a hot bath and then your feet. The temperature of the water may be bearable for

LEFT AND RIGHT SIDES
If you drew a line down the centre of your body from top to bottom, everything on the right half of your body would correspond to the reflex points on the right foot and hand, while everything on the left half of the body would correspond with the left foot and hand. Keep this image in mind to help you locate and remember the different reflex points.

your hands but it will probably be too hot for your feet. The reflexes on the hands are harder to isolate than they are on the feet, as the surface area of the hands is much smaller. However, often it is more practical to work on the hands: you can give yourself a discreet treatment at work, whereas with a foot treatment you need to ask a friend or partner to treat you. For this reason a hand treatment is ideal for self-help. Spoil yourself with a complete foot session when you get home at night or are relaxing at the weekend.

ENERGY ZONES

It is easier to understand how reflexology works if you are familiar with the five pairs of longitudinal energy zones, or paths of energy, in the body. These are numbered one to five on either side of the spine and begin in the hands and feet and continue up to the head. The first zonal pair starts in the big toes and runs up the inside of the legs and the spine to the centre of the brain. On the hands, it begins at the tip of the thumbs and continues up the outside of the arms and shoulders to the centre of the neck. Here it joins the pair that started in the big toes.

Reflexologists believe that any condition interrupting the flow of energy through a given zone will disturb the healthy functioning of the body parts lying along it. For the first zonal pair this would include the spine, neck, and brain. In the same way, when you apply pressure to the hands and feet the whole zone will be stimulated and its healing effect felt throughout the body.

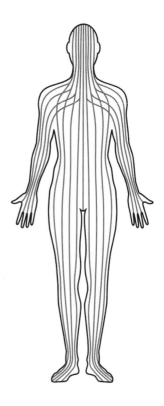

MAPPING THE ZONES
The body is divided into ten energy zones, five on each side of the spine. The zones run from the toes and then up through the head, with zone 1 starting at the big toe. The hands also form part of the zone map, with zone 1 starting at the thumb.

Working guidelines

The divisions of the hands and feet act as guidelines for identifying which areas of the hands and feet relate to which area of the body (see right and below). All reflex points are found within these guidelines (see pp.26-33 for maps of the hands and feet which shows the reflex points).

THE DIAPHRAGM LINE (A)
The foot diaphragm line runs along the top of the metatarsal bones where they meet the toes. It is easy to identify as the skin just above it is darker. On the hands it runs just below the knuckle bones. Reflexes relating to the heart and lungs lie above this line.

THE WAIST LINE (B)
On the foot, run your finger down the outside until you feel a bony protrusion about midway and draw an imaginary line across. The hand waist line runs across the palm where the thumb joins the hand. Reflexes for the digestive system, kidneys, and spleen lie between the waist and diaphragm lines.

THE PELVIC LINE (C)
To find the pelvic line on the foot, draw an imaginary line from ankle bone to ankle bone across the base of the heel. On the hands it starts where the hand joins the wrist.

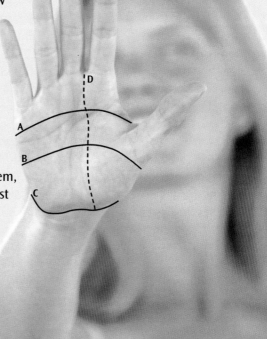

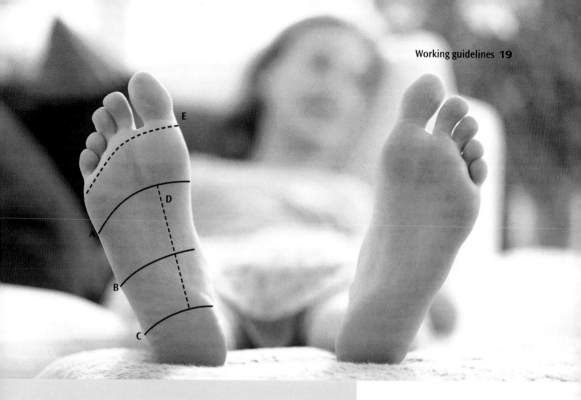

Reflex points for the organs of elimination lie between the pelvic and waist lines. Below it are reflexes for the reproductive organs.

THE LIGAMENT LINE (D)
If you retract the toes to stretch the foot, you will feel a fibrous, elastic-like tendon on the arch between the diaphragm and waist lines. This is the ligament line, which starts on the diaphragm line below the first and second toes and continues down to the pelvic line. On the hands, it starts below the second and third fingers.

THE SHOULDER LINE (E, FEET ONLY)
This line is a secondary guideline for the feet only and runs just below the base of the toes. Above it lie all the reflexes for the sinuses, eyes, ears, thyroid, and neck.

LOCATING THE GUIDELINES
The working guidelines will help you locate the different reflexes on the hands and feet. Because the hands are much smaller than the feet, the hand guidelines are closer together than the foot guidelines. In the same way, the reflex areas on the hands are concentrated in a smaller area and are therefore less detailed (compare foot and hand maps on pp.26–33).

Getting started

Before you begin a reflexology treatment you need to be familiar with a few basic techniques and know how to support the hands and feet when you are working on them. You must also be sensitive to the amount of pressure you use.

If you have time, begin any reflexology session with relaxation exercises (see p.38 and pp.86–9), which are calming and help you "tune in" to the hands or feet you are treating. Equally, it is important to keep your nails clean and short—you should not be able to see them when you look at your hand palm up.

TECHNIQUES

There are four basic reflexology techniques you need to learn, namely creeping, hooking out, rotating, and

CREEPING *(01–04)*
The forward-creeping motion of this technique is similar to how a caterpillar moves. Keep your thumb (or finger) flexed and work with the flat pad, pressing down slightly on the outer edge so that the nail does not dig in. It is a tiny action that lets you work slowly and methodically. Try imagining that you are working on a pincushion full of pins: each time you lift the thumb, creep forward, and press down as if you were pressing in one of the pins.

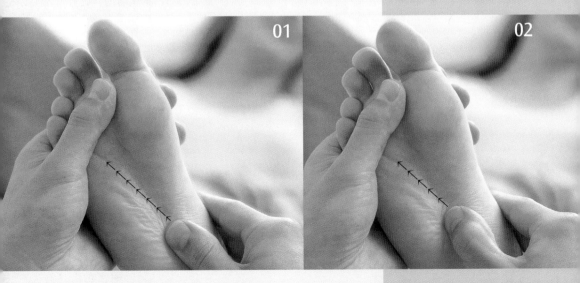

01

02

spinal friction. Experiment on yourself or a friend until the techniques become familiar.

PRESSURE

Some people like a lot of pressure, while others prefer a lighter touch. How much pressure you use is largely intuitive, but generally a healthy person will enjoy more pressure than someone who is elderly or infirm. You need to exert enough pressure for the receiver to feel a reaction in the reflex points, but never apply such force that it causes pain. Bear in mind that when you start giving reflexology it takes time to maintain constant levels of sufficient pressure, as your thumbs and fingers are not accustomed to working in this way.

RIGHT THEN LEFT

Always work the reflexes on the right foot or hand first and complete the entire sequence before treating the left foot or hand. This is so you work with the natural flow of the intestines (see pp.26–33).

Unless otherwise stated, work each reflex area twice, first in one direction and then the other.

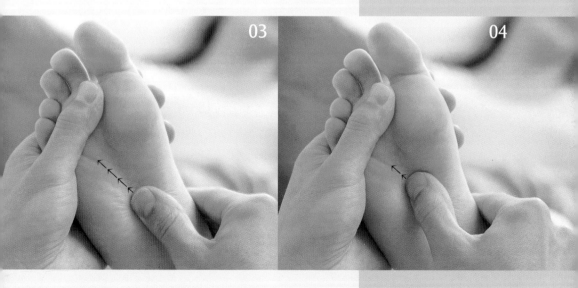

03 04

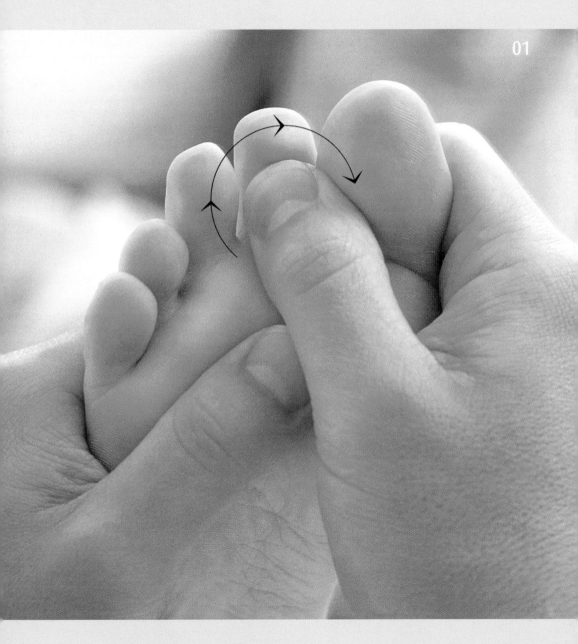

ROTATING *(01)*
When the kidney, adrenal, eye, and ear reflex points need extra stimulation, use the rotating technique.

Place the flat of your thumb on the appropriate reflex point and rotate it inwards, towards the spine, using a small but firm movement. Maintain pressure for several seconds for maximum benefit.

SPINAL FRICTION *(02–03)*
There is a special spinal friction technique for stimulating and warming the spinal column. Place the palm of your hand on the inside edge of the foot or hand (in line with the big toe or thumb) and vigorously rub up and down that area.

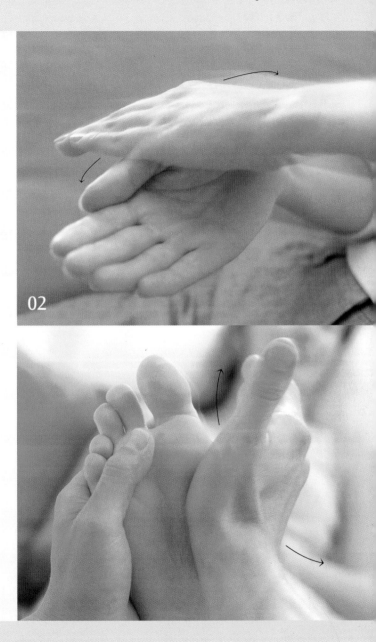

02

SUPPORTING THE FEET
(01–02)
When you work reflex points above the waist line (see p.18), support the top of the foot (01); to work reflex points below the waist line, support the heel (02). This enables you to handle the feet more easily and also helps the receiver relax as they feel more secure.

If you are working the right foot (02), hold it with the left hand and rotate inwards with the right hand. For the left foot, support it with your right hand and rotate inwards with your left. Always rotate the foot inwards towards the spine.

SUPPORTING THE HANDS
For self-help, you can simply hold the hand you are treating with your working hand (see pp.38–9) or rest it in your lap. For added support, rest the hand you intend to treat on a sweater, cushion, or towel.

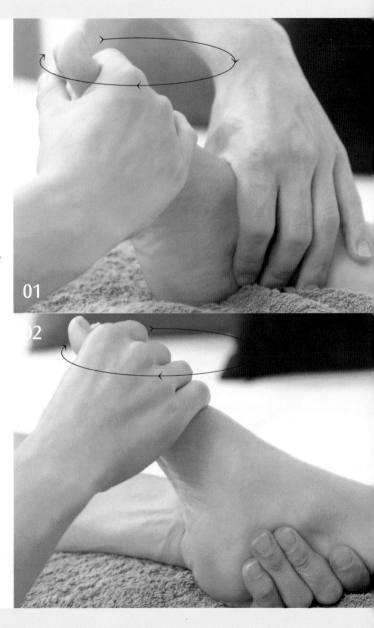

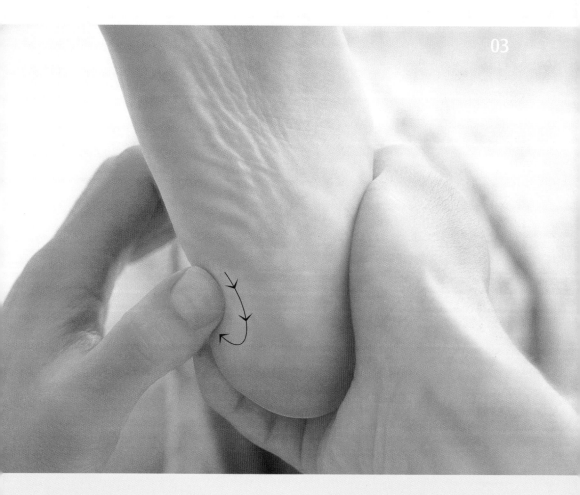

03

HOOKING OUT *(03)*
Use the hooking-out technique to work the ileocecal valve reflex (see p.26), which is located near the pelvic line on the lateral edge of the right hand or foot. The ileocecal valve joins the large and small intestines.

Press down firmly on this point with your left thumb and then use the flat of your thumb to make an outward-hooking movement in the shape of the letter "J". Working this point encourages general elimination and improves bowel function.

The feet: soles

The following maps of the feet and hands group together the many thousands of reflexes according to which body part they affect. Each area mapped, for example the heart, stomach, or spleen, contains many reflex points, rather like pins on a pincushion. However, in the interest of clarity the individual areas will be referred to in the singular as the heart reflex, stomach reflex, etc. These areas also overlap, so when you work one area you will often contact reflex points for another.

MIRRORS OF THE BODY

Use these maps to help you locate all the reflex points. You will see that the feet and hands truly do mirror the rest of the body. For example, the spleen is located in the upper left abdomen behind the ribs and the corresponding reflex is located on the outer edge of the left foot and hand. It is also interesting to note that the shape of the spinal reflex on the inner edge of the feet resembles the curved shape of the actual spine.

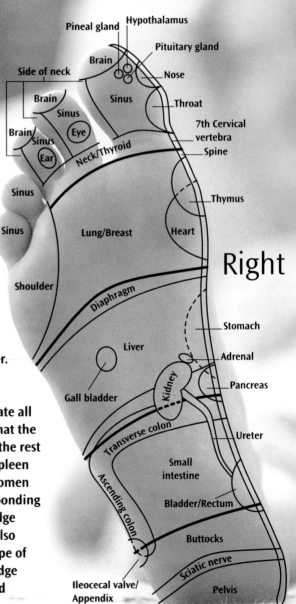

Pineal gland
Hypothalamus
Pituitary gland
Brain
Nose
Side of neck
Brain
Sinus
Throat
Brain
Sinus
Eye
7th Cervical vertebra
Brain
Sinus
Ear
Neck/Thyroid
Spine
Sinus
Sinus
Lung/Breast
Heart
Thymus
Shoulder
Diaphragm
Right
Stomach
Liver
Adrenal
Kidney
Pancreas
Gall bladder
Transverse colon
Ureter
Small intestine
Ascending colon
Bladder/Rectum
Buttocks
Sciatic nerve
Ileocecal valve/ Appendix
Pelvis

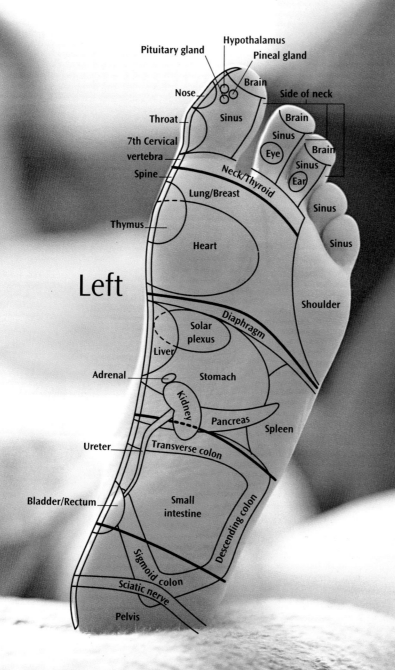

Pituitary gland

Hypothalamus

Pineal gland

Brain

Nose

Side of neck

Throat

Sinus

Brain

7th Cervical vertebra

Sinus

Eye

Brain

Spine

Neck/Thyroid

Sinus

Lung/Breast

Ear

Thymus

Sinus

Heart

Sinus

Left

Shoulder

Diaphragm

Solar plexus

Liver

Adrenal

Stomach

Kidney

Pancreas

Spleen

Ureter

Transverse colon

Bladder/Rectum

Small intestine

Descending colon

Sigmoid colon

Sciatic nerve

Pelvis

The feet: tops and sides

There are fewer reflexes on the tops and sides of the feet, so these maps are much simpler. This is because the tops of the feet are too bony to allow effective contact to the reflexes.

Note the positions of the knee and hip reflexes. This is an isolated instance of the reflex points not mirroring the body.

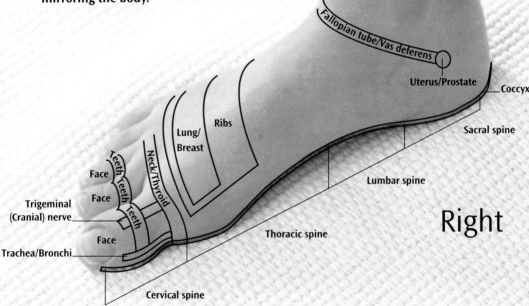

Fallopian tube/Vas deferens

Uterus/Prostate

Coccyx

Sacral spine

Ribs

Lung/Breast

Lumbar spine

Neck/Thyroid

Teeth Teeth Teeth

Face

Face

Face

Trigeminal (Cranial) nerve

Trachea/Bronchi

Thoracic spine

Right

Cervical spine

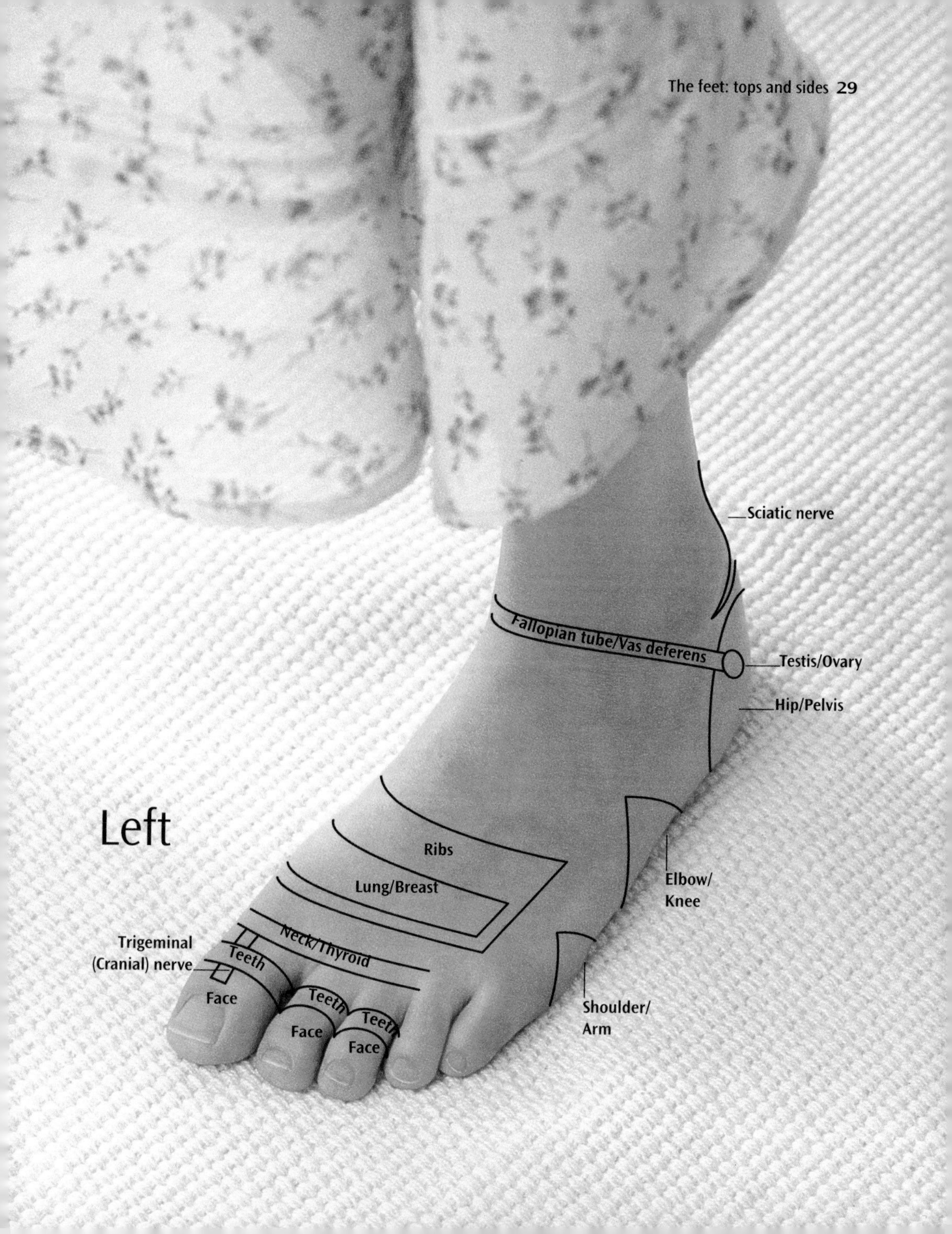

Sciatic nerve

Fallopian tube/Vas deferens

Testis/Ovary

Hip/Pelvis

Left

Ribs

Lung/Breast

Elbow/
Knee

Neck/Thyroid

Trigeminal
(Cranial) nerve

Teeth

Face

Teeth

Teeth

Face

Face

Shoulder/
Arm

The hands: palms

Because the hands are much smaller, the hand reflexes are condensed and less obvious than those on the feet. This is one of the reasons why a foot treatment is more effective than a hand treatment (see also pp.16–17).

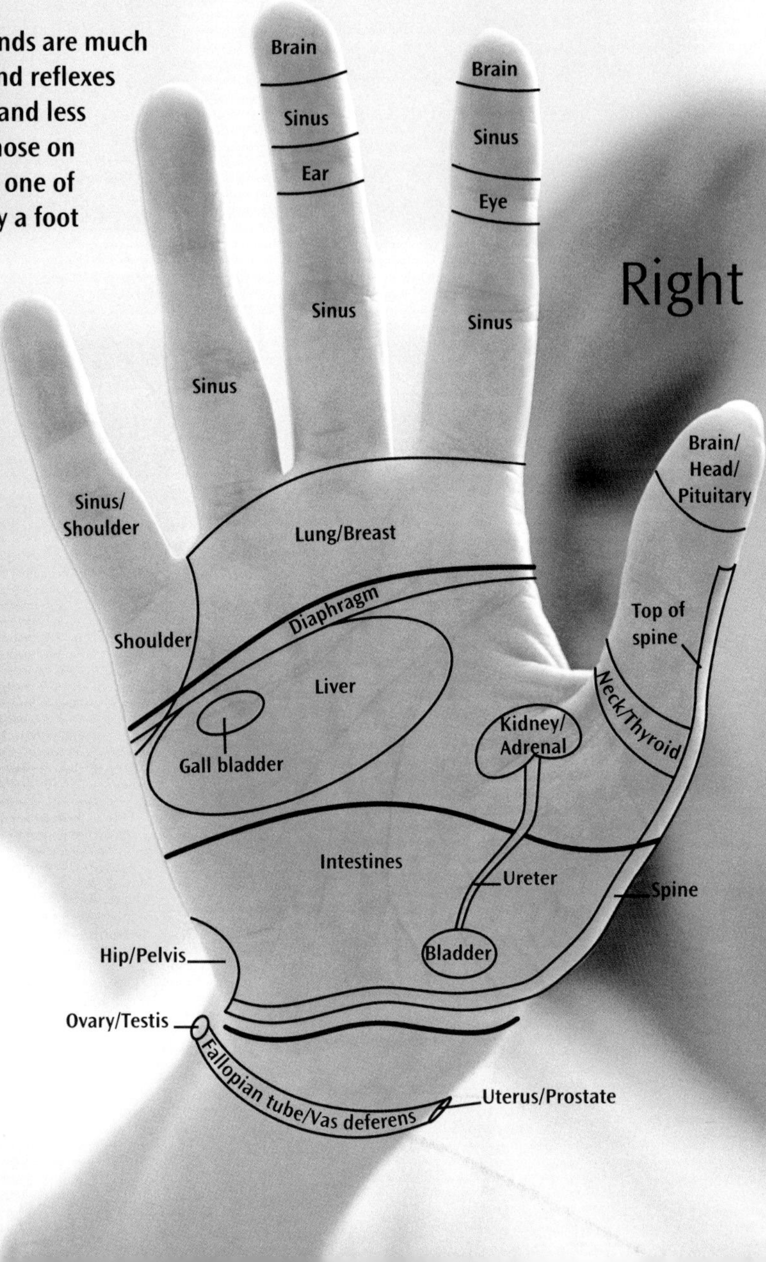

Brain

Brain

Sinus

Sinus

Ear

Eye

Right

Sinus

Sinus

Sinus

Sinus

Brain/
Head/
Pituitary

Sinus/
Shoulder

Lung/Breast

Top of
spine

Shoulder

Diaphragm

Neck/Thyroid

Liver

Kidney/
Adrenal

Gall bladder

Intestines

Ureter

Spine

Hip/Pelvis

Bladder

Ovary/Testis

Fallopian tube/Vas deferens

Uterus/Prostate

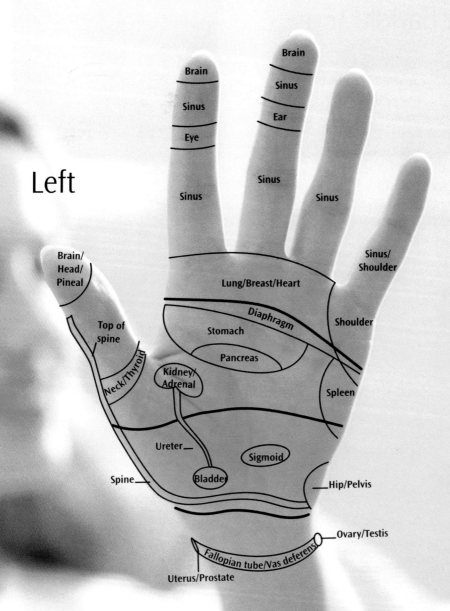

Left

The hands: tops

Because the tops of the hands are too bony to contact reflexes effectively, large areas have been left unmapped.

Note how some of the reflexes, such as the ear, eye, and vas deferens/fallopian tube reflexes, continue all the way around the wrists and fingers to form bracelets.

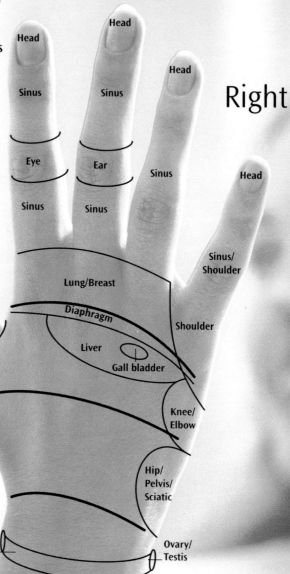

Right

Head
Head
Head
Head
Sinus
Sinus
Sinus
Eye
Ear
Sinus
Sinus/Shoulder
Sinus
Sinus
Lung/Breast
Diaphragm
Shoulder
Thyroid
Liver
Gall bladder
Knee/Elbow
Hip/Pelvis/Sciatic
Uterus/Prostate
Fallopian tube/Vas deferens/Groin lymph
Ovary/Testis

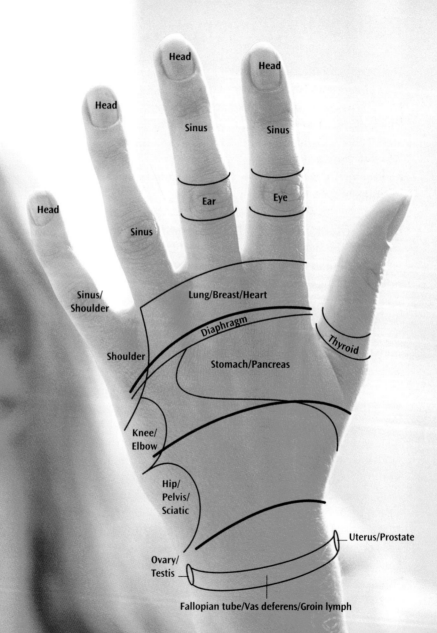

Left

Head

Head

Head

Head

Sinus

Sinus

Sinus

Ear

Eye

Sinus/
Shoulder

Lung/Breast/Heart

Diaphragm

Thyroid

Shoulder

Stomach/Pancreas

Knee/
Elbow

Hip/
Pelvis/
Sciatic

Uterus/Prostate

Ovary/
Testis

Fallopian tube/Vas deferens/Groin lymph

Reflexology everywhere

The beauty of reflexology is that it is easy to use in most environments and without any specialist equipment. For self-treatment, all you need are your hands. However, you may wish to support your hands in your lap with a folded-up sweater, cushion, or towel. Whether you are at home, at work, or on a train, hand treatments are quick and easy to give to yourself at any time of day.

GIVING AND RECEIVING FOOT TREATMENTS

For maximum benefit, foot reflexology should be given by another person to allow the healing energy released during the treatment to freely circulate in the body. Take it in turns with a friend or partner to give and receive treatments. Because it takes a little longer for a foot session, it is best to set aside time together in the evenings or at weekends. Sharing quality time with a loved one in this way is a healing experience in itself, and you will be amazed at how much comfort you can draw from the physical contact alone.

The receiver should sit in a comfortable armchair, resting their legs in an elevated position on a low stool or dining chair, and their feet on a large cushion in the giver's lap. Use a soothing foot moisturizer or balm—peppermint is particularly invigorating—to soften the feet, as this will make it easier for the giver to work over the feet with the thumb (if the foot is very dry it will be harder to work the reflexes). However, only use a little moisturizer and avoid massage oils altogether as it is very hard to contact the reflexes properly on slippery skin.

HOW OFTEN IS ENOUGH?

Young or old, how often you have reflexology depends on whether you are trying to treat a recurring problem or simply wish to maintain your state of health. It also depends on how much time you have. For example, if you suffer from a condition such as constipation, indigestion, migraine, or back pain, you should aim to have a full foot treatment two or three times a week and supplement each treatment with regular hand sessions. Even the most chronic health conditions can respond to reflexology treatment sessions, often when all else has failed. If, however, you are fit and healthy and just want to use reflexology to stay that way, a full foot session on a monthly basis is usually enough, interspersed with occasional hand treatments.

READY FOR TREATMENT

Once you are familiar with the four basic reflexology techniques and feel comfortable with the different ways of supporting the hands and feet, you will be ready to give reflexology at any time. Initially you may need to refer back to these pages and you will almost certainly need to consult the foot and hand maps on pp.26–33, which show you how the different parts of the body correspond to the various reflexes on the feet and hands.

Now you have all the information you need to treat either yourself or another person, read on to see how easy it is to fit reflexology into your day as part of a stress-free and healthy lifestyle.

CHAPTER TWO

Preparing for the day

How do you feel when you open your eyes to
another day? Do you yawn, stretch your body,
wriggle your toes, and have that glad-to-be-alive
feeling, or do you long to pull the
duvet back over your head and hide away
from the world?

Instead of sleeping until the last minute, set aside enough time to prepare yourself mentally and physically for the day ahead. This will help you enter the day in a positive frame of mind and pave the way to a happier and stress-free lifestyle.

If you want to get off to a good start, the secret is not to rush first thing in the morning. Give yourself time for a ten-minute reflexology routine, a leisurely shower, and a sensible breakfast, all of which will prepare you, body and mind, for the day ahead.

As you emerge from bed, stretch your body, press your toes downwards, raise your arms above your head, and rotate your wrists and ankles. Relax your jaw and take some slow, deep breaths, inhaling through your nose and exhaling through your mouth. Concentrate on your chest rising and falling. A deep breath is like a gift to every cell in your body: it aids your circulatory system, your brain, and your muscles. It is very difficult to feel tense and anxious if you breathe slowly and deeply. Deep, conscious breathing slows the heartbeat, reduces anxiety, and lowers blood pressure. It also helps the body burn up waste products and release endorphins, the body's natural analgesic. With controlled, rhythmical breathing you can bring yourself into harmony with the world.

After a few minutes, stand next to your bed, touch your toes, and rotate your hips. When you take a shower, finish off with a cool rinse to stimulate your circulation.

Reflexology to start the day

Reflexology is a great way to get your blood circulating and your energy flowing first thing in the morning. These quick hand exercises are easy to perform on yourself and will stimulate your entire nervous system. Follow the complete sequence of exercises on the right hand before treating the left hand.

Picture 01 shows you properly how to warm up your hands and is a vital part of all self-help hand exercises. The hand moulding exercise is a good all-round relaxation technique, while the diaphragm relaxation exercise is excellent for relaxing the respiratory system, as it helps to relax the diaphragm muscle at the base of the lung. Use the creeping technique on pp.20–1 for the diaphragm relaxation exercise as well as to work the lung reflex on the palms and tops of your hands.

REFLEXOLOGY

Warm-up: spinal friction *(01)*
Rub the outside edge of your thumb with your other palm.

Hand moulding *(02)*
Knead your palm with the fist of your other hand.

Diaphragm relax *(03)*
Creep your thumb along the diaphragm line.

Lung reflex *(04–05)*
Work the lung (04) from the diaphragm line to the base of the fingers, then work down the lung reflex on top of your hand (05).

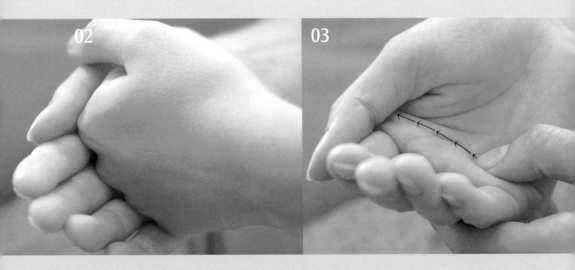

02

03

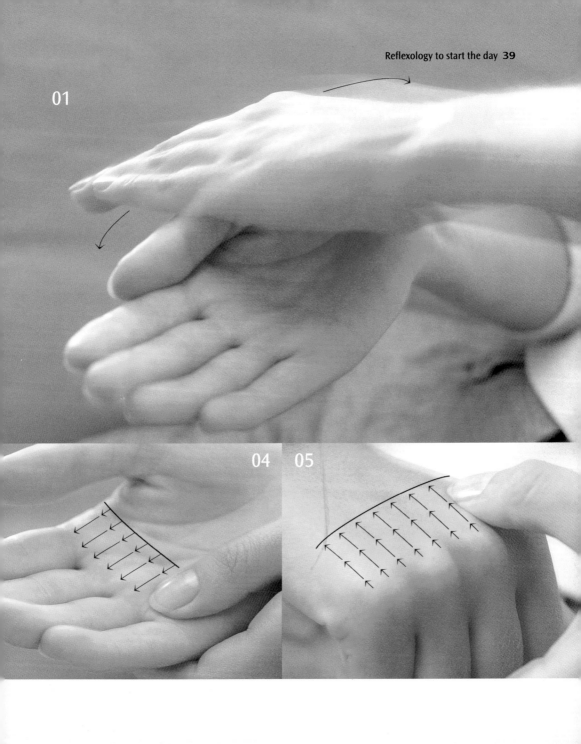

Energy breakfasts

A quick reflexology treatment will give you an energy boost, but you must also eat a nourishing breakfast to activate your metabolism after the long fast of the night. If you do not replenish your blood sugar levels you will soon feel lethargic, find it harder to concentrate, and be easily irritated.

You can prepare a healthy breakfast in just a few minutes. Be inspired by the ideas right and below for a tasty and nutritious start to the day. Avoid coffee as it can make you tense and anxious; instead, try drinking Caro, Barleycup, or dandelion coffee.

FIVE-MINUTE BREAKFASTS
A combination of any of the following will see you through the morning.

Oatmeal porridge and milk sweetened with chopped dried fruit, such as apricots and cranberries. This is ideal for cold winter mornings.

A poached egg (you can poach an egg in a microwave oven in a few seconds) on a slice of wholemeal toast.

A variety of fresh fruit, such as fresh apricots, grapes, and watermelon. You could also add a spoonful of plain, live yoghurt.

Instead of coffee or ordinary tea, try a mixture of dried red clover, nettle, and lemon balm, shown here with a sprig of fresh lemon balm. Not only does it taste great but it also helps flush out any toxins.

Alternatively, try a fresh fruit shake (not shown). Pour one large glass of apple juice into a liquidizer and add a chopped banana and pear. Liquidize the contents and drink. This is ideal if you find it hard to get·up in time to prepare a proper breakfast.

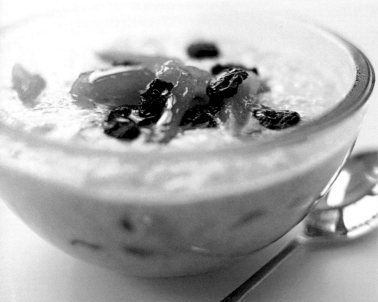

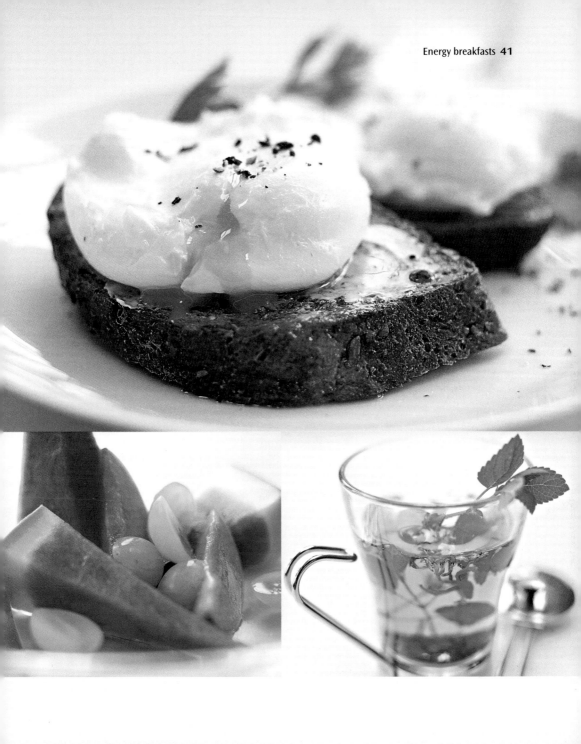

Throw off a cold

If you wake up with a headache, streaming nose and eyes, and a sore throat you have probably caught a cold. Reflexology can greatly alleviate the symptoms, although use only the relaxation exercises on p.38 if you have a fever. Follow the entire routine on your right hand and then work the left. Do the warming up exercises on p.38 before you start.

GENERAL SELF-HELP
Many home remedies also help you overcome a cold:

■ Add the juice of a freshly squeezed lemon and 2 tsps of honey to a mug of hot water.

■ If your nose and sinuses are blocked, prepare an inhalation. Add five drops of one of wintergreen, juniper, or peppermint essential oils to a bowl of hot water. Leaning over the bowl, place a towel over your head, and breathe slowly but steadily.

■ To boost your immune system, take 10 drops of echinacea tincture two or three times a day and 500mg of vitamin C once a day.

■ Drink at least 2 litres (4 pints) of water during the day to flush out your system. It will also replenish bodily fluids—few people realize that a runny nose has a dehydrating effect on the body.

■ Honey works wonders on an irritating cough. For a calming drink, mix 2 tsps each of honey and apple cider vinegar in 30ml (½ pint) of warm water. Alternatively, 1 tsp of freshly chopped thyme in honey will soothe the throat and chest and act as an expectorant.

■ Suck a zinc lozenge every three hours to calm a sore throat or cough and boost your immune system.

REFLEXOLOGY

Throat (01)
Creep all the way around the base of the thumb.

Face & Sinuses (02)
Creep up each of the fingers in turn, starting at the base of the little finger.

Spine (03)
Creep your working thumb along the top of the pelvic line and up the outside edge of the thumb.

Spleen (04)
The spleen reflex is below the diaphragm line and on the outside edge of the left hand only. However, creep across the entire palm as shown.

Brain (05)
Apply firm pressure to the top of your thumb with the thumb of your other hand.

Eye & Ear (06)
Hold the eye reflex, under the first bend of the index finger. Work it using the rotating technique. Repeat on the ear reflex, which is just below the first bend of your middle finger.

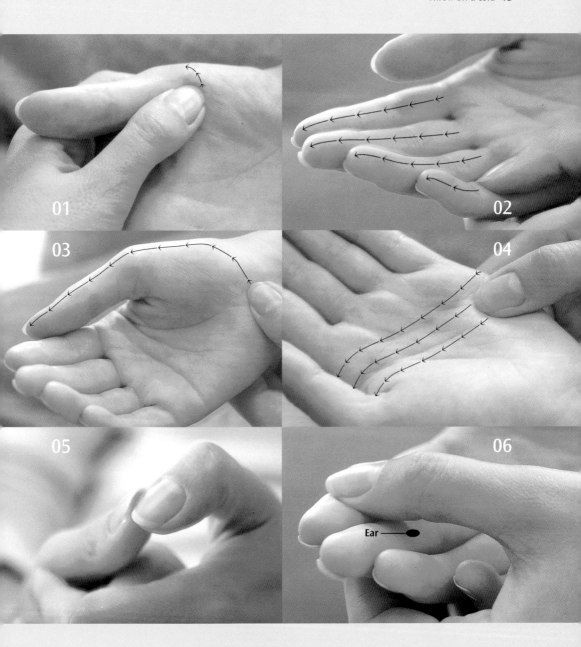

01

02

03

04

05

06

Ear

Headache solutions

You can wake up with a headache for a multitude of reasons, including dehydration, a cold (see p.42), flu (see pp.128–9), low blood sugar level, stress, tiredness, or eye strain (see p.73). Resist hiding it with painkillers and instead remove the cause and therefore the pain (to treat migraine, see pp.74–5).

Reflexology brings immediate relief to a headache, particularly if you have time for a foot treatment (see pp.122–3). However, this self-help hand treatment is almost as effective.

GENERAL SELF-HELP

■ Drink plenty of pure water to rehydrate the body and flush out impurities, and cut out any foods that may aggravate the symptoms, such as coffee, black tea, cheese, milk, chocolate, and alcohol.

■ If you are very tired, try to sleep more. See pp.106–7 if you are having problems sleeping.

■ Regular headaches can be a sign of bad eyesight, so visit your optician.

■ A teaspoon of honey restores your blood sugar level.

■ Relax in a warm bath having added five drops of one of lavender, peppermint, or marjoram essential oils.

■ Apply a cold compress (see opposite) using rose essential oil.

■ Ask your partner to give you a head, neck, and shoulder massage (see p.101), adding a few drops of peppermint or aniseed essential oil to your carrier oil. If symptoms persist, take a small pot of tiger balm with you into the office. Use it to gently massage your forehead, sinuses, and temples during a quiet moment.

REFLEXOLOGY
Work all the reflexes on the right hand first and then work the left. Before you begin, warm up the hand you are treating (see p.38).

Brain (01)
To work the brain reflex point, apply firm pressure to the top of your thumb with the thumb of your other hand.

Spine (02)
The spine reflex begins at the base of the hand and continues up the outside edge of the thumb. Work along the entire reflex using the creeping technique to relieve tension in the vertebral column and central nervous system.

HANGOVER HEADACHES
Some headaches are self-induced if you have drunk alcohol in excess, in which case you should also work the liver reflex (see pp.64–5).

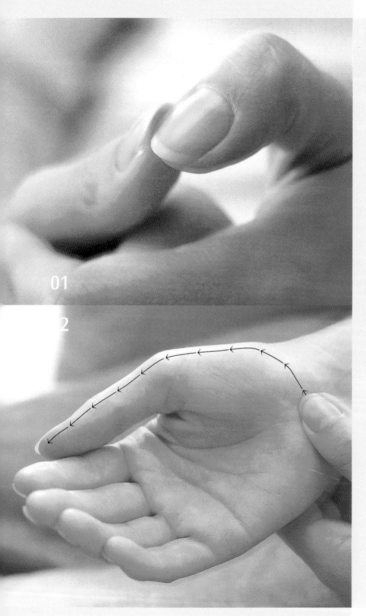

01

2

GENERAL SELF-HELP
Avoid taking aspirin, which can irritate the stomach, and resist coffee, as this will further dehydrate you. Instead, drink plenty of water throughout the day to flush out the system and replenish fluids.

After treating your hands, lie on your bed with a cold compress for 10 minutes. To prepare it, put six ice cubes in 100ml (1 pint) of water and add five drops of one of rose, geranium, or chamomile essential oils. Soak cotton-wool pads in the solution and lay them on your temples and forehead.

Try eating a slice of dry rye toast or a small bowl of plain, live yoghurt and honey topped with oats or wheatgerm. If, however, you feel nauseous, just sip a cup of peppermint tea.

Tackling period pains

Painful periods, with or without heavy bleeding, are miserable. Sometimes constipation is the cause, as a congested bowel puts pressure on the uterus. Eat a balanced diet (see pp.102–3) to keep you regular and be careful of what you eat the week before your period (see right). Take plenty of gentle exercise: yoga, swimming, and walking are particularly good for preventing and relieving painful periods.

Reflexology also brings rapid relief from painful periods. If the symptoms are severe, ask someone to work your feet (see pp.134–5). For self-help, work each hand in turn, as shown below, using the creeping technique. See p.38 for warming-up exercises.

BEFORE YOUR PERIOD

■ *Drink plenty of water.*
■ *Eat more wholegrains, such as brown rice and pasta, oats, and granary bread.*
■ *Eat more phytoestrogens, such as chickpeas and soya.*
■ *Eat more linoleic acid. This is found in linseed, soya, and sunflower and sesame seeds.*
■ *Eat calcium in green vegetables (e.g. parsley, watercress, or broccoli), chickpeas, beans, and lentils.*

REFLEXOLOGY

Uterus *(01)*
Work the uterus with the middle finger of your other hand. The uterus reflex is on your wrist below the thumb.

Ovary *(02)*
Use the same finger to work the ovary reflex on the inside edge of the hand, in front of the wrist bone.

Fallopian tube *(03)*
Use all four fingers of your working hand to contact this reflex, which encircles the wrist like a bracelet.

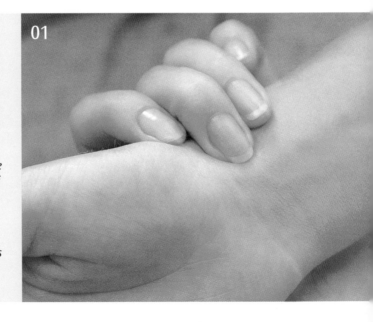

01

GENERAL SELF-HELP
■ Add a couple of drops of chamomile essential oil to a carrier oil, such as almond oil, and gently massage into the abdomen.
■ To relieve uterine cramping take dong quai, a traditional herbal remedy, in capsule form.
■ Sipping chamomile tea counteracts pain and nervous tension. Raspberry leaf tea reduces bloating.
■ Relax in a warm bath, adding five drops of one of Roman chamomile, marjoram, or cypress essential oils to help abdominal cramps.
■ Lie with a well-wrapped hot water bottle on your abdominal area or lower back to relieve cramping.

BEFORE YOUR PERIOD
■ *Cut out or reduce caffeine: drink no more than three cups a day.*
■ *Cut down on all protein.*
■ *Reduce foods containing refined sugar.*
■ *Drink alcohol in moderation only.*

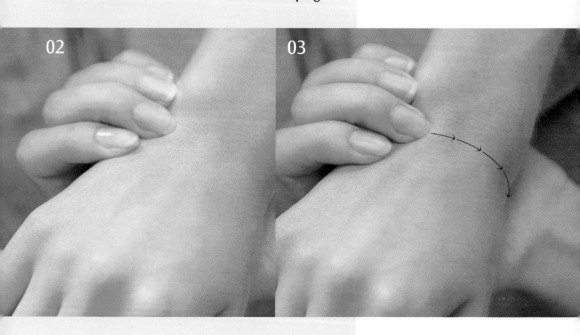

Morning sickness

Many women suffer from morning sickness, generally unpleasant and inconvenient, during the first 12 weeks of pregnancy. During early pregnancy the body produces an excess of female hormones to stabilize the foetus in the uterus. This causes extra fluid to circulate in the brain and affects the balancing mechanisms in the inner ear—like motion sickness.

Reflexology helps, especially if the pituitary gland and the entire digestive system are worked on the feet. However, if you are on the train and feel a wave of nausea, work the hands as shown.

GENERAL SELF-HELP

■ Don't get out of bed too quickly. Take a cup of sweet tea or peppermint tea with a dry biscuit before you rise.
■ Avoid bending over from the waist, as this can irritate the vagus nerve. Instead, squat down, which also stretches the lower back and opens the pelvis.
■ Put a few drops of ambrette seed essential oil on a tissue and inhale slowly and deeply. This is an ideal way to combat nausea if you are travelling or at work.
■ Suck slippery elm tablets, drink ginger tea, or nibble ginger biscuits.
■ Watch your diet, as a deficiency of certain vitamins seems to aggravate morning sickness, notably zinc and vitamin B complex. Zinc is found in red meat, pumpkin seeds, and green vegetables, while bananas, basil, and ginger are good sources of vitamin B6.
■ Low blood sugar may be a contributory factor, so try eating a protein-rich snack half an hour before going to bed. Eating little and often seems to help, too.

REFLEXOLOGY

Brain (01)
After warming up the hand you intend to treat (see p.38), apply firm pressure to the top of your thumb with the thumb of your other hand.

Neck & Thyroid (02)
Work all the way round the base of the thumb using the creeping technique.

Adrenal (03)
Contact the area shown on the fleshy part of the hand using the creeping technique. For extra stimulation use a deep rotation on the area indicated.

Pancreas, Stomach, & Spleen (04)
The pancreas, stomach, and spleen reflexes are on the left hand only. Creep across the area as shown.

CAUTION
Seek medical advice if vomiting is severe and does not abate. If you have a history of miscarriage, do not attempt any of the reflexology exercises.

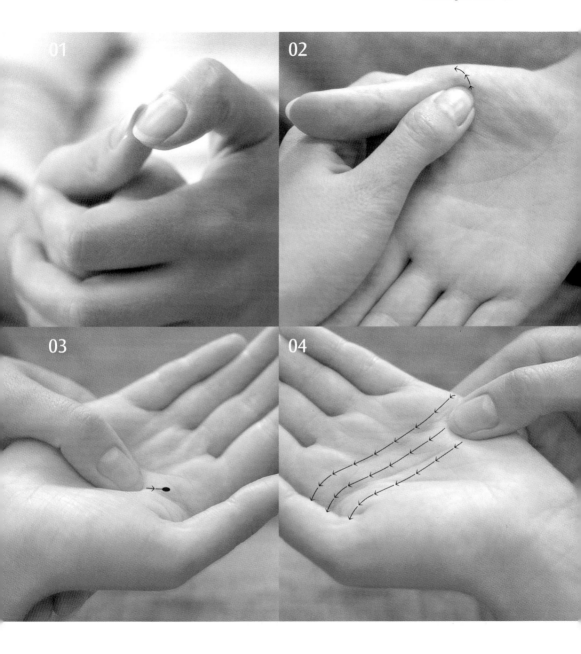

CHAPTER THREE

Travel in balance & harmony

With increasingly sophisticated travel systems, it is becoming ever easier to travel long distances, either for work or for leisure. Although it may be easier to travel, it is also more stressful, as there are more people on the move, customer expectation is higher, and everybody has less time on their hands.

Whatever means of transport you use, travelling can test the mildest of tempers. Fortunately, there are many things you can do to make your journey as comfortable and as relaxing as possible. Reflexology is a very useful tool to keep you calm in stressful situations or to give you an energy boost and encourage good circulation on long-distance journeys. The beauty of it is that you only need your hands and a little know-how.

If you travel in the morning, make sure you eat a nourishing breakfast (see pp.40–1) and avoid coffee: caffeine stimulates the adrenals and makes you tense. Be aware of what you eat *en route* and avoid salty snacks or junk food: salt encourages water retention and can make your feet, legs, and ankles swell and eyes puffy. Instead, prepare a travel picnic with a large bottle of water, a banana for energy and concentration, and a small but nutritious bag of sunflower and pumpkin seeds.

On long journeys, particularly by air (see pp.56–9), wear flat shoes and loose-fitting clothing as tight waistbands and trousers restrict breathing and circulation.

If you drive regularly use a backrest for added support and comfort, as sitting in a fixed position for any length of time stresses the lumbar spine and can lead to back problems. Take regular breaks if you drive for long distances. This restores concentration and lets you stretch out tension held in the body, particularly in the hip and spine muscles.

Panic attacks

Panic attacks are terrifying and can strike without apparent provocation or reason, although frequent sufferers often identify certain circumstances that bring them on, such as travelling by public transport or shopping. As unpleasant and as frightening as they may be, you must remember that the attack will pass, either in a few seconds or a few minutes. See pp.132–3 for longer-term treatment.

COPING WITH AN ATTACK: GENERAL SELF-HELP
Wherever you are there are many things you can do to control or cope with an attack.
- Draw slow, deep breaths, resting your hand on your

GENERAL SYMPTOMS
The first time you have a panic attack you might think you are having a heart attack, are about to die, or are going mad. It is common to feel faint, short of breath, nauseous, to sweat, have hot or cold flushes, need to go to the bathroom, or feel pains or discomfort in your chest.

Do not feel alone if you suffer from panic attacks, as around 35% of people have at least one in their lives.

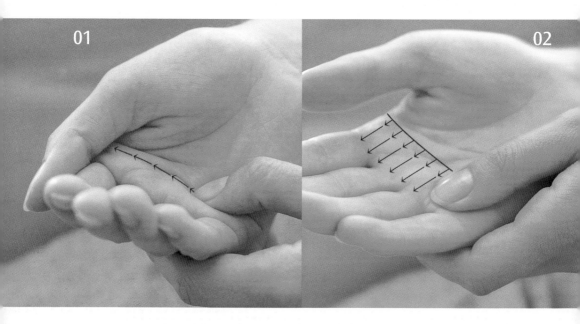

REFLEXOLOGY

A simple hand treatment when you start to feel anxious will help you relax and often ward off an attack altogether. It also diverts your attention from your anxiety and lets you take control of the situation.

Use the creeping technique to concentrate on the easy-to-find diaphragm and lung areas. When you feel calmer, work the entire hand methodically (see pp.60–7).

Diaphragm (01)
Work your thumb along the diaphragm line from the inside to outside edge.

Lung: palms (02)
Work the lung reflex on the palm of your hand from the diaphragm line to the base of the fingers.

Lung: top of hands (03)
Work down the lung reflex on the top of your hand using your thumb or index finger.

stomach and feeling it rise and fall. If you hyper-ventilate, try breathing slowly and steadily into a paper bag. This reduces the amount of oxygen and increases the levels of carbon dioxide in your blood.

■ Divert your attention by focusing on banal tasks or objects, such as what you need to buy for dinner.

■ If you can, get up and walk or jog around to burn off excess adrenalin. You can be discreet about this by pretending to go to the bathroom.

■ Many people find that a few drops of Bach Flower Rescue Remedy work wonders.

■ Try listening to soothing music or meditations on a personal stereo to avoid becoming over-anxious.

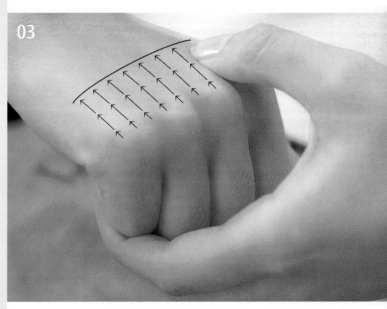

03

Travel sickness

While some people can sail on the roughest of seas with little or no reaction, others only have to sit in a moving car to feel nauseous, faint, and start vomiting. Travel sickness is caused by an oversensitivity of the inner ear, which affects the body's balance and in turn the stomach. Reflexology is an effective antidote to travel sickness, and the simple hand treatment below will alleviate the symptoms and restore the body's balance. Treat the right hand first and then the left.

GENERAL SELF-HELP
With a little thought and preparation you can make any journey more comfortable.

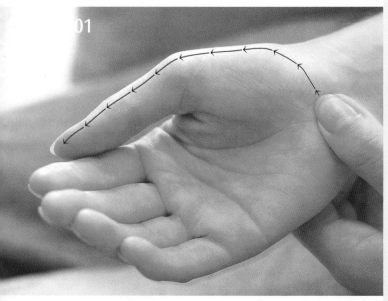

01

REFLEXOLOGY
Start by warming up the hand to be treated (see p.38) and then work the reflexes indicated.

Spine *(01)*
Work all the way along the spine reflex as shown. Because the spine incorporates the central nervous system, this will help balance the entire body.

Sinuses *(02)*
Use the creeping technique to treat the sinus area. Work up each of the fingers in turn, starting at the base of the little finger. The little finger is also the reflex for the shoulder, which overlaps the sinus reflex.

Ear *(03)*
Apply pressure to the ear reflex point with the thumb of your other hand and use a deep rotation three or four times. The reflex point for the ear is located just below the first joint of the middle finger.

■ Don't be tempted to eat any rich or spicy food the night before your journey. Eat one or two slices of dry toast before you leave and do not take caffeine in any form before or during your trip.

■ Drink ginger tea, nibble on ginger biscuits, or take ginger capsules to combat nausea and alleviate gastrointestinal distress. If you don't care for ginger, suck a piece of fresh lemon or peppermint sweets.

■ Face the direction of travel and, if you are in a car or coach, sit at the front. Make sure the vehicle is well ventilated. If you are travelling by sea, stand outside and take slow, deep breaths of fresh sea air while focusing on the horizon.

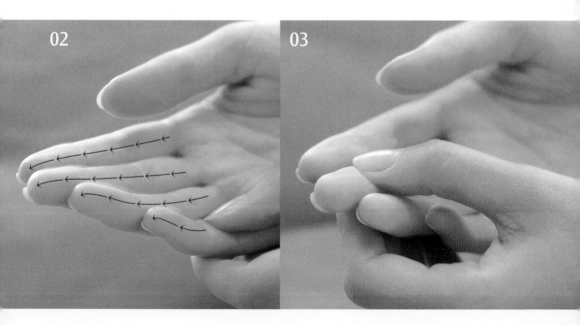

Flying

Travelling by aeroplane is often the fastest and most convenient way to reach a destination, so more and more of us are taking to the skies for business and pleasure. Despite the glamour and excitement associated with air travel, it is often an extremely tiring experience. Use reflexology and the general self-help advice to minimize the side effects of air travel and make your journey more comfortable.

BOOST YOUR IMMUNE SYSTEM

Breathing dry, recycled cabin air challenges the strongest of immune systems, particularly if you are already tired: not only do passengers share each other's germs and viruses for hours, but the body's natural filters—the nose, throat, lungs, and eyes—get

KEEP HYDRATED

The simplest yet most important thing you can do is to drink plenty of water to replenish lost fluids from breathing the extremely dry cabin air. Although alcohol may help you relax, it is well worth resisting that complementary glass as it is a diuretic and therefore encourages dehydration. Instead, choose mineral water. It is also worth taking your own 2 litre (3½ pint) bottle to top up your glass.

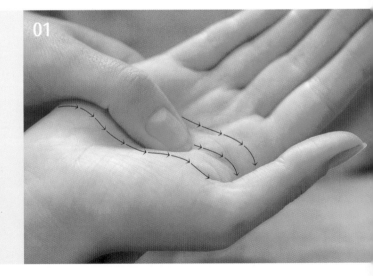

REFLEXOLOGY

Liver *(01)*
The liver reflex is located on the right hand only. You will find it between the diaphragm and waist lines and stretching across the palm from the little finger to the middle finger.

Use your left thumb to creep across the entire area shown, which will also contact the intestines. Work this area three or four times.

dry and cannot work as efficiently. Reflexology is excellent for boosting the immune system and will help your body fight off infections. For best results, follow the complete hand treatment on pp.60–7 and spend a few extra minutes working the liver and spleen reflexes as shown here.

GENERAL SELF-HELP
- Avoid any salty snacks (see p.51).
- If you have dry skin, take a mister with you and spray your face at regular intervals.
- Take vitamin C, which is also a great anti-inflammatory, or tincture of echinacea before you fly. Zinc is also good for the immune system while vitamin B complex will help you cope with stress.

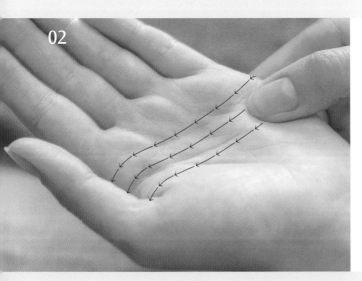

02

Spleen (02)
The actual spleen reflex is on the outer edge of the left hand only. It lies below the little finger and under the diaphragm line. It finishes just below the waist line.

Use your right thumb to creep across the entire area illustrated, not just the spleen. This will also contact the reflexes for the stomach, pancreas, and intestines. Repeat three or four times.

GUARD AGAINST DEEP-VEIN THROMBOSIS

Even if you can indulge in the luxury of business or first class seats, you must move regularly to protect your circulation. Movement also prevents backache and general stiffness. Although the heart pumps blood around the body, it also relies on the body's momentum to help pump blood to the extremities. When you remain still for long periods of time, your circulation slows and blood can stagnate in parts of the body, particularly in the legs, and form clots. This is known as deep-vein thrombosis, which can be fatal if the clot is circulated to the heart or brain. To guard against deep-vein thrombosis give yourself the full reflexology hand treatment during your flight, as shown on pp.60–7.

GENERAL SELF-HELP

There are many general precautions you can take before and during your journey to protect your circulation.

■ Take garlic tablets before you start your journey and then seven hours later. Garlic helps to thin the blood and encourages good circulation.

■ Wear loose and comfortable clothing (see p.51).

■ When seated, rotate your feet at regular intervals. Press them down to the floor and then upwards to the ceiling. Take a few deep breaths or yawn.

■ Make sure you get up every couple of hours and walk from one end of the plane to the other. Raise yourself up on to your toes and then back on your heels so you feel a pressure and stretching sensation in your calves.

ARRIVING AND BEATING JET LAG

When you arrive at your destination take a shower as soon as possible. Rinse your legs and feet thoroughly with cold water to stimulate your circulation and help any swelling in your feet and legs, then if possible lie down for half an hour with your legs well elevated.

The most common after-effect associated with long-haul flights is jet lag, as changing time zones disrupts the body's clock. Generally, the more hours you spend in the air, particularly if you travel eastwards, the longer it takes to recover. Being unable to sleep or needing to sleep at strange hours can leave you feeling anxious, confused, or even depressed for several days.

GENERAL SELF-HELP

■ Once you reach your destination, encourage your body to fall in with the new time zone. If you arrive during the day when normally you would be sleeping, walk around outside and stay awake until evening. If you arrive at night when normally you would be awake, close all the curtains and lie down and rest. Sprinkle a few drops of lavender oil on a tissue and lay it on your pillow. You will probably drift off and actually sleep quite deeply. This will help normalize the body's natural secretions of melatonin, which helps it prepare for sleep.

■ Valerian drunk as a tea or in capsule form has a sedative effect on the nervous system. It helps dispel nervous tension and promotes sound sleep.

■ If you feel out of sorts and are having difficulties sleeping, try taking lecithin.

MELATONIN

Melatonin is a hormone-like substance that helps regulate the body's internal clock. It is secreted by the pineal, a small, pea-sized gland at the base of the brain that responds to changing levels of light. When it is dark more melatonin is secreted and when it is light production stops. Too little melatonin causes sleeping difficulties (see pp.106–7), while too much often leads to depression (see pp.116–17).

Complete hand treatment

The following pages show a complete reflexology hand treatment, which should take you about 25 minutes. Work all of the reflexes on the right hand first and then repeat the treatment on the left. Don't forget to warm up the hand you intend to treat (see p.38).

Ideally, when treating a condition, you should try to give yourself a full hand treatment and then spend more time on the appropriate reflexes for that condition. However, because time is often short this is not always possible. Long journeys are the perfect opportunity for a complete treatment. Not only will it pass away the time, but it will also stimulate your circulation and prevent tension from building up in the neck, shoulders, spine, and hips if you have to sit in the same position for any length of time.

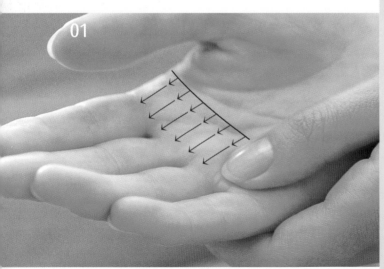

REFLEXOLOGY

Lung: palm *(01)*
Work the lung reflex on the palm of your hand from the diaphragm line to the base of the fingers.

Lung: top of hand *(02)*
Work down the lung reflex on the top of your hand using your thumb or index finger.

Sinuses *(03)*
Use the creeping technique to treat the sinus area. Start at the base of the little finger and work up each of the fingers in turn.

Eye *(04)*
The eye reflex is located just below the first bend of your index finger. Use the thumb of your working hand to apply a deep rotation three or four times.

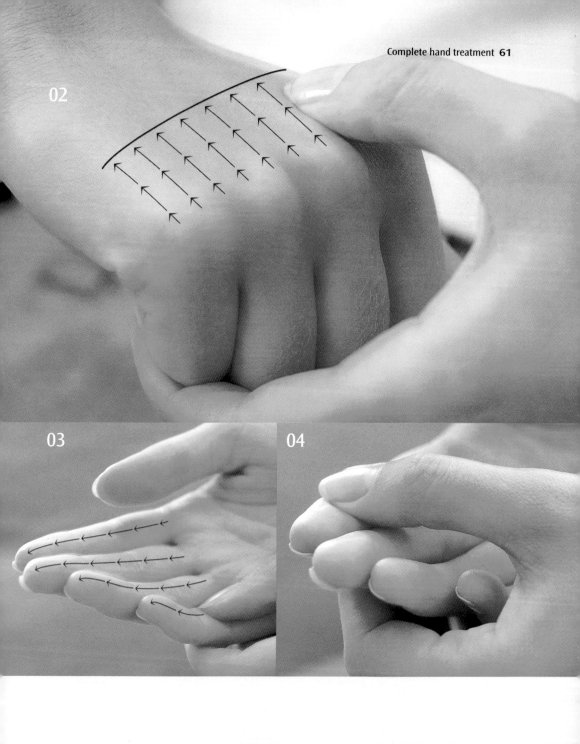

02

03

04

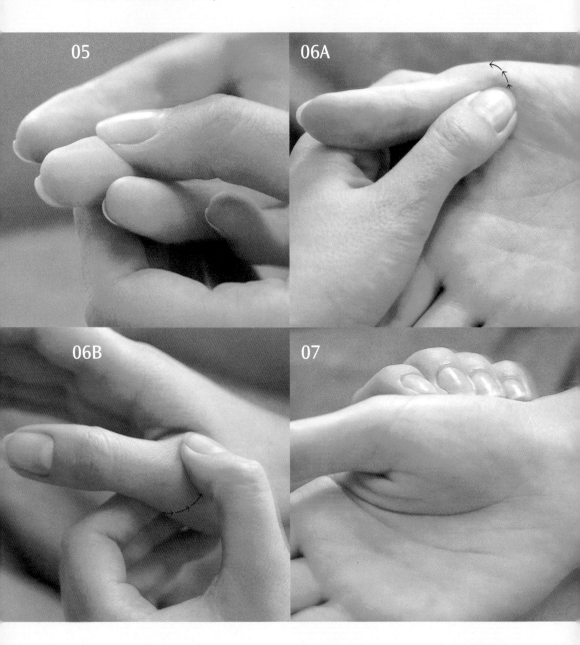

Ear *(05)*
The reflex point for the ear is located below the first joint of the middle finger on either hand. Use your working thumb to apply a deep rotation three or four times.

Neck & Thyroid *(06, A & B)*
Work the base of the thumb (06, A) and continue all the way around it (06, B) using the creeping technique.

Coccyx *(07)*
The coccyx reflex lies at the base of the spine. Apply firm pressure with the four fingers of your working hand.

Hip, Pelvis, & Sciatic *(08)*
The hip, pelvis, and sciatic reflex points are located on top of the hands below the little finger. To contact this area, apply pressure with your four working fingers to the outside edge of the hand you are treating.

Spine *(09)*
Creep along the entire spinal reflex from the base of the hand and up the outside edge of the thumb.

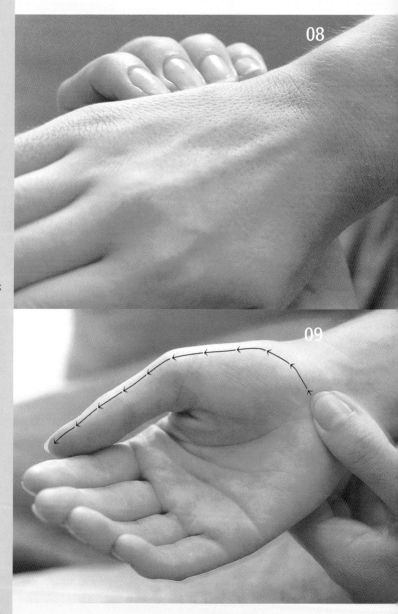

08

09

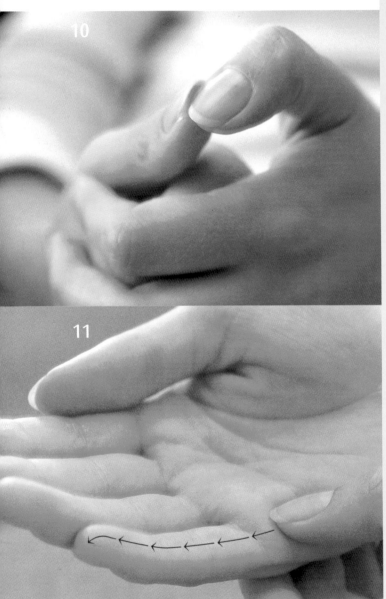

Brain (10)
Apply firm pressure to the top of your thumb with your working thumb.

Shoulder (11)
Use your thumb to creep up the little finger from the diaphragm line. This reflex overlaps the sinus area.

Knee & Elbow (12)
This small, triangular-shaped reflex point is on top of the hand, below the little finger. It sits between the diaphragm and waist lines. Creep across this area with your working fingers.

Stomach area (13)
Creep your thumb across the palm of your left hand only, to contact the stomach, pancreas, and spleen.

Intestines (14, A & B)
Creep across your palms as shown. On the right hand (14, R) you will work the liver, gall bladder, ileocecal valve, and ascending and transverse colon, while on the left hand (14, L) you will contact reflex points for the transverse, descending, and sigmoid colon.

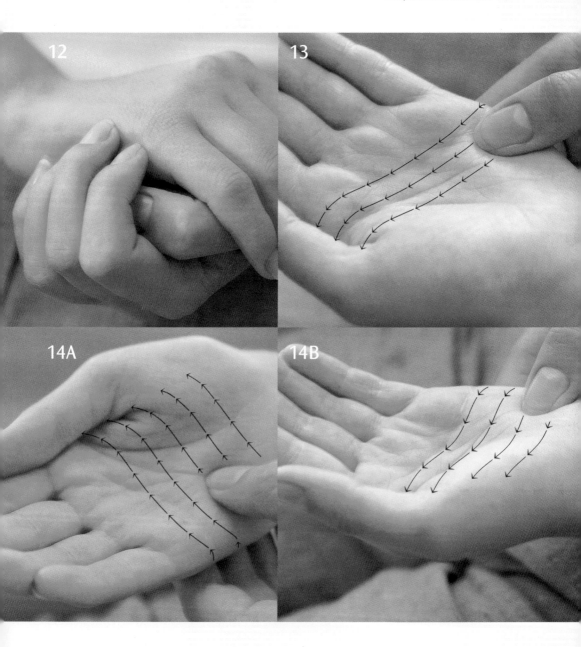

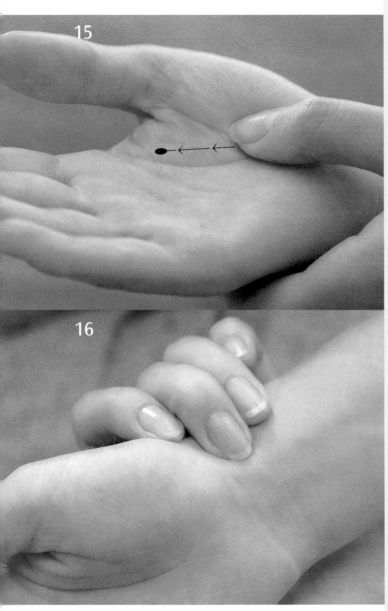

Urinary system (15)

The urinary system comprises the bladder, ureter tube, and kidney reflexes.

To contact reflexes for the bladder, work up the fleshy part of the thumb using the creeping technique. Continue up the hand towards the base of your index finger, which will also work the ureter tube.

The kidney reflex is above the ureter tube. Carry on working up the fleshy part of the thumb until you reach the diaphragm line. Apply a deep rotation to this area to work the kidney. You will also contact the adrenal, which sits on top of the kidney inside the lateral line.

Uterus/Prostate (16)

You will find the uterus/prostate reflex on the outside edge of your wrist, below the thumb. Contact this area by applying pressure with the middle finger of your working hand.

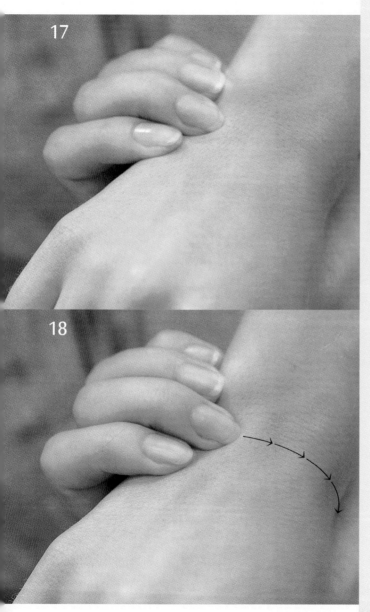

Ovary/Testis *(17)*

Use the same finger to work the ovary/testis reflex on the inside edge of the hand, below the little finger and in front of the wrist bone.

Fallopian tube/Vas Deferens *(18)*

These reflex points encircle the wrist like a bracelet. When you have worked the ovary/testis continue all the way around your wrist to contact the fallopian tube/vas deferens using all four fingers of your working hand.

CHAPTER FOUR

Staying on top at work

Even if you are cool and collected when you arrive at the office, it is often hard to remain unruffled by the demands of your job: flurries of emails, faxes, and telephone calls all vie for your attention, while meetings with colleagues and clients can take up the entire morning.

Try to arrive at the office early so you can plan your day and open your mail uninterrupted. Avoid taking any calls and treat this time as your own. Being prepared makes you feel calm, confident, in control, and therefore more likely to be successful. However, if you are still nervous about a business appointment, calm yourself with the reflexology treatment on pp.52–3.

Pay attention to your personal workspace as you subconsciously respond to your environment, which can affect your concentration and productivity. Keep your desk surface clean and clutter-free and file or throw away anything you are not working on or no longer need. Piles of messy papers make you look and feel disorganized, as well as trap energy. At the end of the day, spend a few moments tidying your desk and filing your work so that you are greeted by a fresh space of possibilities the next morning.

Many modern offices are air-conditioned and rely heavily on artificial lighting, particularly in windowless rooms, thus depriving you of fresh air and natural light. To immediately improve the atmosphere, arrange a vase of fresh, sweet-smelling flowers, such as freesias, on your desk. Try also to spend time outside every day, particularly in the morning or at lunchtime: artificial lighting does not reproduce the full spectrum of light present in daylight and therefore cannot stimulate the pineal gland as effectively (see p.59). This can cause headaches, migraine, or even depression.

Protecting posture

Most people spend their working day slouched at their desk in front of a computer. Bad posture stresses the neck and back, particularly the lumbar spine. It also hinders breathing as it compresses your chest cavity and makes it harder for the lungs to function efficiently.

When you are at your desk, sit with your computer directly in front of you so you are not twisting your body to view the screen. Your monitor should be at eye level or just below eye level, otherwise you will strain your neck and develop headaches from staring upwards at the screen. Take care to adjust your chair properly so that your feet are flat on the floor and your thighs are at right angles to your body (use a foot stool if necessary). Resist crossing your legs as this both twists the hips and spine and restricts the supply of blood to the legs. Ensure the small of your back is properly supported and use a small cushion or rolled-up towel if you need extra support. Hold your head upright with your shoulders back and down in a relaxed manner. Keep your back upright and, when you lean forwards, do so only from the waist. Place the keyboard to the front of your desk and when you type keep your elbows at 90 degrees to your body. Your wrists should be flat and in a straight line. Move the mouse with your whole arm and avoid bending your wrist sideways.

Check your posture regularly and shift your position to avoid tension building up in any part of your body. The strong muscles in your shoulders can suffer from repeated and long periods of work on a keyboard. If, however, you do develop back or neck pain, follow the reflexology treatment on p.72.

STRETCH AND MOVE
No matter how busy you are it is vital that you get up at least once an hour to move your body and stretch your limbs. This will relieve any tension held in the body and encourage good circulation: blood can stagnate in your extremities if you stay still for any length of time (see p.58).

Repetitive strain injury

Repetitive strain injury, or RSI, is caused by overuse of the hands, fingers, and wrists, and is common among people who type for long periods of time. Heavy lifting exacerbates the condition. Symptoms include tingling, aching, a burning sensation, swelling, and a numb sensation in the fingers, hands, wrists, or arms. The pain can also spread to the neck and shoulders. Women who are pregnant or menopausal are more likely to suffer from RSI, as changes in the hormonal system create an excess of fluids, which congest the ligaments, in particular the densely packed wrist ligaments.

At first sign of any problem you must rest the hands and wrists and apply ice packs. If you ignore the early symptoms you will permanently damage your ligaments. Rest your wrists on two small packets of frozen peas, and remain in this position for at least 10 minutes. Refreeze the packs and repeat the process three or four times throughout the day. Acupuncture is also very beneficial and helps to heal the inflammation in the tendons. Always seek relief from complementary therapies before considering surgery.

However, try to prevent the problem from occurring altogether by sitting at your desk properly (see left), taking regular breaks from typing to exercise your hands and wrists (see right), and giving yourself regular, full reflexology treatments as shown on pp.60–7.

PREVENTIVE EXERCISES
Protect yourself from RSI by taking regular breaks from typing and following these simple but effective exercises.

Rotate your shoulders and bend your neck forwards, backwards, and side to side.

Put an elastic band over your fingers and thumb and gently flex them.

Drop your arms by your sides and gently shake your wrists and arms.

Sitting upright in your chair, clasp your hands and bring them straight up over your head. Ease them backwards to stretch your shoulders and upper back.

Hold one arm out in front of you with your hand palm up. Grasping the fingers with your other hand, bend the wrist back as if you were trying to touch the top of your forearm with the back of your fingers. Repeat on the other hand.

Back and neck pain

Often, despite taking precautions, you can still suffer from back or neck pain, particularly if you are stressed, as the tension in your mind can manifest itself in your neck and shoulders. Taking five to ten minutes to give yourself a hand reflexology treatment will bring great relief, both to the pain and to the tension in your mind. Work each hand in turn, although be sure to first warm up the hand you intend to treat (see p.38).

At such times deep breathing will help dispel tension held in the body. Close your eyes and take slow, deep breaths. With each exhalation imagine your worries leaving your body and feel your shoulders, neck, and jaw becoming heavy and relaxed.

REFLEXOLOGY
Spine & Neck (01)
Creep along the entire spinal reflex as shown. Work the area twice then creep all the way around the base of the thumb to contact the neck.

Shoulder (02)
To contact the shoulder, use your thumb or index finger in a creeping motion to work from the diaphragm line up the whole length of the little finger.

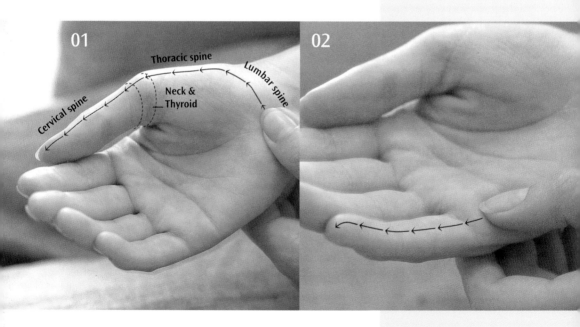

01
Thoracic spine
Lumbar spine
Neck & Thyroid
Cervical spine

02

Eye strain

Staring fixedly at a VDU screen for hours often causes eye strain and headaches (see also pp.44–5). If you feel tension around your temples, press them with your index fingers and apply a deep rotation until the muscles around your eyes and sides of your face relax.

GENERAL SELF-HELP (SEE ALSO PP.112–13)

■ Don't look at your computer screen for longer than 20 minutes without a break. Exercise and relax your eyes by looking out the window or not focusing at all.
■ Consciously relax your facial muscles when you look at the screen, particularly around the eyes and forehead.
■ Carry a bottle of eye drops for immediate eye relief.

REFLEXOLOGY
Sinuses (01)
After warming up the hand, start at the base of the little finger and work up each of the fingers in turn using the creeping technique.

Eyes (02)
Next use the thumb of your working hand to apply a deep rotation three or four times to the first bend of your index finger. Repeat the sequence on your other hand.

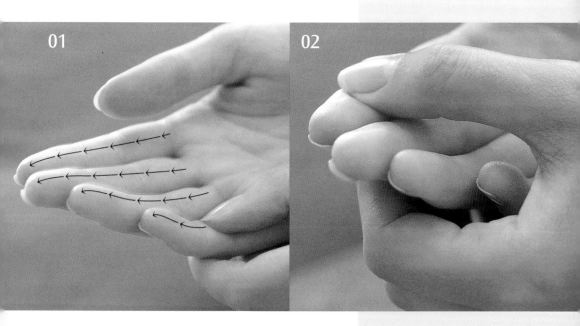

Migraine

A migraine is not just a headache but a totally disabling condition causing severe head pain, blurring of vision, and repeated attacks of nausea. Migraine is strongly linked to the digestive system and is often an adverse reaction to a food or foods. Many high fat foods, such as chocolate and cheese, trigger an attack.

As with all illnesses, there is never one single cause but a combination of several: an extremely stressful day at work may bring on a migraine yet not be the root cause of the problem.

Reflexology can bring considerable relief to migraine, particularly if you treat the feet. If possible, ask a friend or colleague to give you the treatment on pp.122–3, otherwise follow the self-help hand treatment below.

EARLY SYMPTOMS
Symptoms usually begin in childhood, although initially do not often manifest as a headache, but as non-specific symptoms, such as abdominal pains, vomiting, dizziness, or unusually severe motion sickness. Most sufferers have a family history of migraine and incidences usually peak between the ages of 25 and 35 then start to decline.

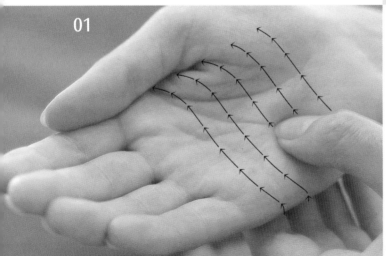

01

REFLEXOLOGY
Right palm (01)
Warm up the right hand (see p.38) and work across the area of palm indicated. Use the creeping technique to contact the reflex points for the liver, gall bladder, right kidney, and intestines, including the ascending and transverse colon and the ileocecal valve.

GENERAL SELF-HELP

■ It is extremely important that you drink plenty of filtered water to flush out the liver.

■ Drink peppermint tea to reduce nausea. For a premenstrual migraine, drink vervain tea.

■ Rub a few drops of lavender essential oil into the temples to relieve tension.

■ Stop what you are doing, close your eyes, and relax, if possible with a basil cold compress (see p.45).

■ Eating cheese, chocolate, red wine, oranges, and food colourings can cause migraine. Try eliminating one or two of these for a couple of weeks to see if there is an improvement in the frequency or severity of your attacks. Wait a further week and eliminate another two items. You will usually find the culprit.

WOMEN AND MIGRAINE

It is quite common for women to suffer migraine prior to their periods, which recede when menstruation begins. This is due to changes in the hormonal system and can also occur during the menopausal years.

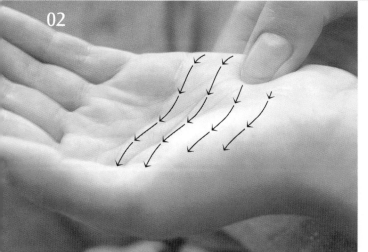

02

Left palm (02)

After warming up the left hand (see p.38), work across the centre of the palm as indicated in a creeping motion. This will contact the reflex points for the stomach, pancreas, left kidney, and intestines, including the transverse, descending, and sigmoid colon.

Energy lunches

What you eat at lunchtime is also important. You need unrefined carbohydrates and some protein, as well as vitamin C and natural sugars in fruit. If possible, avoid eating at your desk, as the change of scene will do you good. If you prefer to go out for lunch, find a salad bar and don't be tempted by rich, heavy, or sugary foods. Fast food is full of empty calories, while sugary soft drinks and alcohol upset blood sugar levels. Alcohol will also make you drowsy.

HEALTHY, EASY LUNCHES
The following suggestions will provide you with all the energy you need for the afternoon and are simple to prepare at home.

A bowl of soup is an excellent winter warmer. Simmer puy lentils together with cubes of potato and carrot in a clear stock. Garnish with fresh basil and slices of red chilli.

Pockets of pitta bread are a tasty alternative to ordinary bread. Try filling them with a mixed bean salad of kidney, broad, green, and butter beans. Top with alfalfa and lettuce.

Rice salads are equally simple to prepare. Add chopped red onion, steamed asparagus, green peppers, and a dash of balsamic vinegar to a mixture of cooked wild and plain rice. Garnish with flat parsley.

A fresh juice, such as the carrot, celery, and apple juice shown here, is a great pick-me-up.

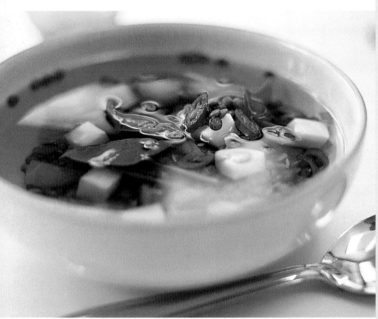

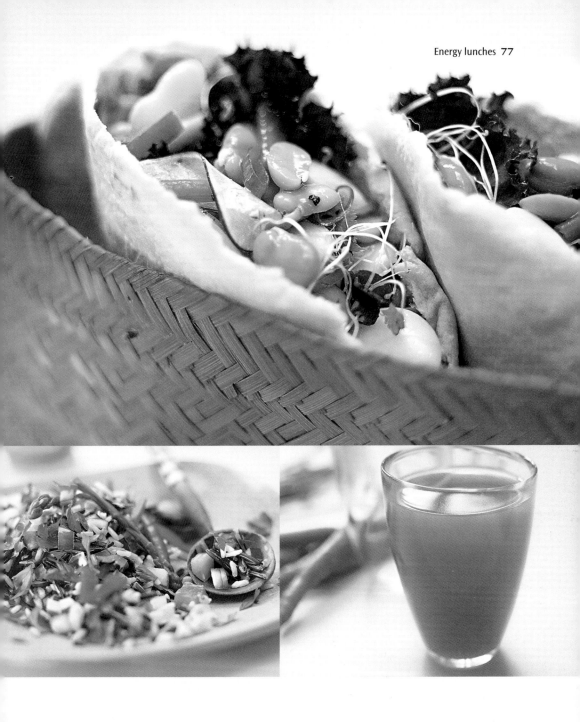

Recharging your batteries

Set aside small amounts of time throughout the day to refocus your mind. When you do, rather than drinking a cup of coffee or lighting a cigarette, spend two or three minutes breathing slowly and deeply (see p.37). Breathing is energizing and relaxes the mind—often the best ideas and most effective solutions come when you stop thinking about a problem.

Taking a proper break for lunch is also essential for replenishing your mental and physical energy. Some people go to the gym or swimming pool for a quick work-out, but if you only have a little time or no facilities available, simply leave the office and go for a brisk walk outside, stopping to do some breathing exercises. If you work near a park, walking under rustling trees and inhaling the cool, fresh smells of greenery lets you forget the morning and restores your

REFLEXOLOGY

Sinuses *(01)*
After warming up the hand you are treating, use the creeping technique to contact the sinus reflex points. Start at the base of the little finger and work up each of the fingers in turn.

Intestines *(02)*
On the right palm, work across the hand to contact the reflexes for the liver, gall bladder, right kidney, and intestines, including the ileocecal valve, ascending and transverse colon.

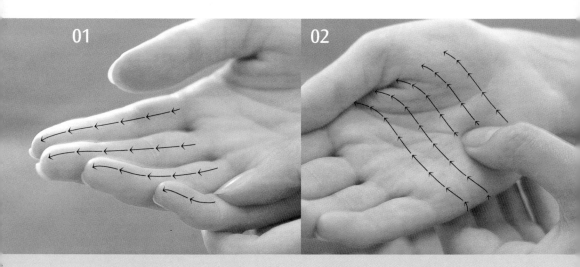

spirits. Even if you only step out for ten minutes, the change of scene, fresh air, and natural light will help you continue working with precision and efficiency.

REFLEXOLOGY FOR ENERGY BOOSTING

Many people have a dip in energy mid-afternoon as they digest. If you need to revive yourself after eating, or indeed at any other time, follow the treatment below. Work the right hand first and then the left.

GENERAL SELF-HELP

■ Make sure your office is well ventilated. Poor air quality often contributes to drowsiness.
■ Inhale a few drops of basil or ginger essential oils on a tissue to clear your head and restore your energy.
■ Drink ginger tea to aid your digestive system.

Intestines (03)
On the left palm, work across the hand as shown to contact the reflexes for the stomach, pancreas, left kidney, and intestines, including the transverse, descending, and sigmoid colon.

Spinal friction (04)
Briskly rub the outside edge of your thumb with the palm of your working hand.

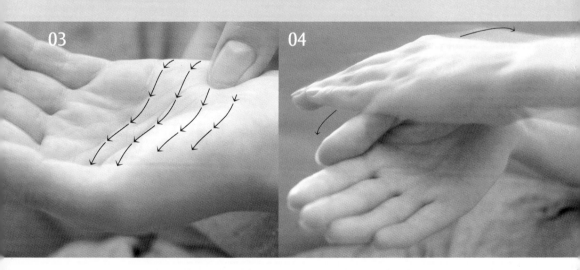

Easing indigestion

If you eat in a hurry or on the move, swallow your food without chewing it properly, or indulge in rich, spicy dishes, you may develop indigestion. Your state of mind and physical well-being also affect your digestion, so if you are anxious, stressed, overworked, or overtired, you will disturb the stomach's gastric secretions and general activity.

Indigestion, or dyspepsia, is a term used for a number of symptoms brought on by eating and processing food, including abdominal discomfort or pain, bloating, excess wind and belching, regurgitation of gastric acid, heartburn, and lack of appetite.

Reflexology can bring quick relief to indigestion. Start by warming up the hand you intend to treat (see p.38) and then work the reflexes shown. When you have completed the sequence on one hand, treat the other.

REFLEXOLOGY
Use the creeping technique to contact all of the reflexes in this sequence.

Sinuses (01)
Work the sinus reflex points. Start at the base of the little finger and work up each of the fingers in turn.

Lung: palms (02)
Work the lung reflex on the palm of your hand from the diaphragm line to the base of the fingers.

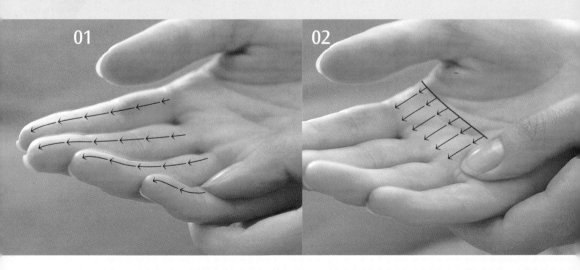

GENERAL SELF-HELP

Preventing indigestion is much better than trying to treat it, so ask yourself what brought it on. Did you eat too quickly or too much? Do certain types of food disagree with you? Are you eating a balanced diet (see pp.102–3)? Are you particularly stressed at work? If you address these questions you should be able to avoid indigestion altogether. To alleviate your current symptoms, try drinking the following, but not for at least half an hour after eating:

- For heartburn, acidity, and dyspepsia, dissolve 1 tsp of bicarbonate of soda into a mug of hot water and sip gradually.
- Drinking barley water will help counteract flatulence as will an infusion of six cloves in a mug of hot water.
- Peppermint tea helps stomach pains and flatulence.

Lung: top of hand *(03)*
Work down the lung reflex on the top of your hand with your thumb or index finger.

Spine *(04)*
To contact the spinal reflex, work from the base of the hand to the top of the outside edge of the thumb as shown.

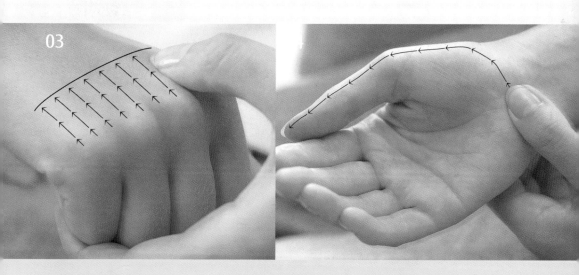

03

Irritable bowel syndrome

If you suffer from irritable bowel syndrome, or IBS, you will probably feel worse after eating, regardless of what and how you have eaten your food. IBS is a common condition of the large intestine and can seriously reduce a person's quality of life. It tends to affect high-striving perfectionists who subject themselves to high levels of stress. What causes IBS is not entirely clear, as there is no evidence of any structural abnormalities of the bowel. However, it has been linked to several dietary and psychological factors. This is perhaps unsurprising, for even people who do not suffer from IBS experience differences in their bowel habits when they are very stressed: nerves can make the bowels rumble and gurgle, become constipated, or loose.

Reflexology brings relief to sufferers of irritable bowel syndrome by improving bowel function and relaxing the overreactive digestive system. For self-help, work the intestinal reflexes on the hands. Follow up this treatment with a foot session when you get home. If symptoms are severe, aim to treat the feet at least three times a week. (For additional general self-help and foot treatment, see pp.130–1.)

GENERAL SELF-HELP
■ A few drops of peppermint oil in a mug of warm water will inhibit gastrointestinal contractions and relieve gas. Peppermint tea is also effective, especially if made with fresh mint.
■ Many plants have a direct antispasmodic action on the gastrointestinal tract, in particular chamomile and

REFLEXOLOGY
Intestines
Start by warming up the right hand (see p.38). Using the creeping movement of your thumb, methodically work across the area of the palm between the diaphragm and pelvic lines to contact all the intestinal reflexes (01). After 2 minutes repeat on the left hand (02).

valerian. These are best taken as a tea, tincture, or in capsule form.

■ Take charcoal tablets for bloating, wind, and diarrhoea.

■ Reassess your diet. Food allergies are closely linked with IBS and wheat and cow's milk are common culprits. Try eliminating products containing one or other for four weeks to see if there is any improvement. At the same time you should also increase your intake of fresh vegetables, fruits, oats, and legumes, which contain water-soluble fibre as well as many other beneficial nutrients.

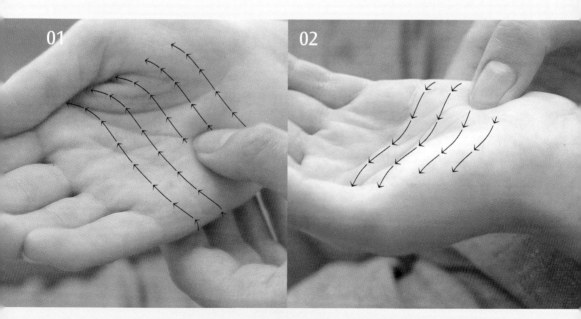

CHAPTER FIVE

Relaxation & recreation

To enjoy time away from work you must be able to unwind completely. Not only will you physically feel better and be less prone to illness but you will also find greater enthusiasm for returning to work and dealing with everyday pressures.

According to Buddhist tradition there are six qualities or virtues a person should have if they are to lead a healthy life, namely patience, optimism, generosity, wisdom, discipline, and stillness. Of these, perhaps stillness is the most important, for great inspiration can be born out of calm. Too often people become irritated, tired, depressed, or ill because they work intensively for weeks without being still.

Evenings and weekends are an ideal time to exchange a relaxing foot treatment with a friend or partner. However, first give yourself time to unwind when you arrive home. The best way to do this is to get into the habit of performing a relaxing ritual, as this signals to your body that it is time to leave behind the day's tensions. Take off your shoes and stretch your arms up and out, breathing slowly and deeply. Next change into some loose clothes, perhaps taking a shower first. Avoid thinking about dinner or opening your mail and just be still for 10 to 20 minutes.

Choose an object that expresses space for you, such as a flower or lit candle, and sit in front of it in a relaxed position. Gaze at it, breathing slowly and deeply. Feel the tension leaving your body with each exhalation. When your mind is still, choose a word that expresses serenity for you, such as peace, calm, or space. As you breathe out, repeat your word. When you are ready, open your eyes, stretch your arms above your head, and slowly stand up. Once your mind is settled continue with the evening.

Complete foot treatment

A full reflexology treatment takes about 45 minutes. Complete the entire sequence on the right foot before treating the left. You treat the right foot first in order to work with the flow of the intestines: the intestines ascend on the right foot and descend on the left.

If you are the receiver, relax in an armchair or recliner with your feet on a large cushion in the giver's lap, who is sitting in front of you (see also pp.34–5). You may wish to receive the treatment in silence, as it is often a great relief to communicate simply by touch after a day of communicating with words. Alternatively, this time is also ideal for catching up with each other's day and sharing any worries.

REFLEXOLOGY
Warming up the foot
Before you begin, apply a little moisturizer to the foot.

Diaphragm relax (01)
Work along the diaphragm line by pressing your thumb into the foot as shown.

Side-to-side relax (02)
Supporting the top of the foot, rock the whole foot from side to side between your palms in a rapid but gentle movement.

Ankle freeing (03)
Support the ankle bones between the fleshy parts of your thumbs. Keeping your wrists loose, gently but rapidly rock the foot from side to side.

Metatarsal kneading (04)
For the right foot, push the fist of your right hand into the sole whilst squeezing the top of the foot with the left—like kneading dough. Change hands for the left foot.

Spinal friction (05)
Use the flat of your hand to vigorously rub up and down the inside of the foot.

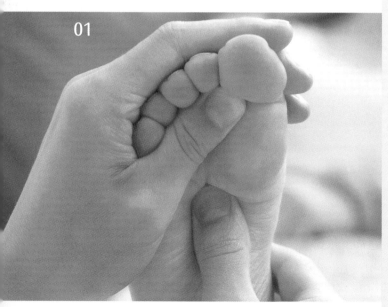

01

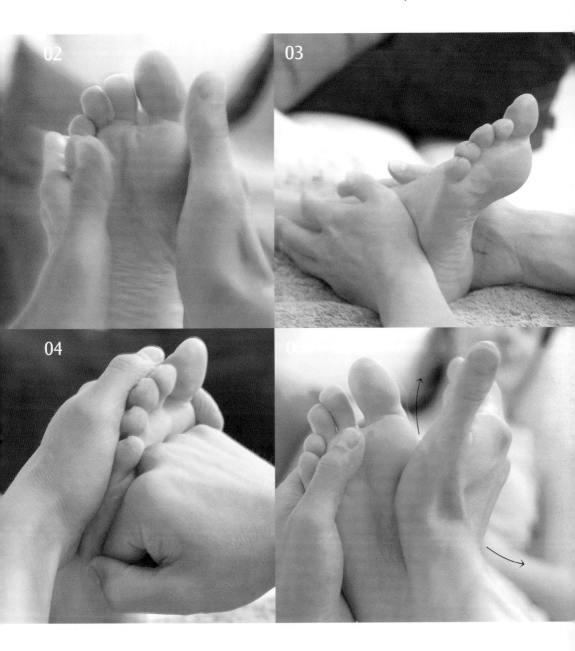

Circling: Overgrip *(05)*

For the right foot, firmly hold the top of the ankle with your left hand as shown and circle the foot inwards and towards the spine with your right.

For the left foot, hold the ankle with your right hand and circle the foot inwards and towards the spine with your left. This exercise will help reduce swollen ankles.

Circling: Undergrip *(06)*

For the right foot, support the heel, as shown, with your left hand and use your right hand to gently circle the foot inwards and towards the spine. Reverse the hand positions on the left foot.

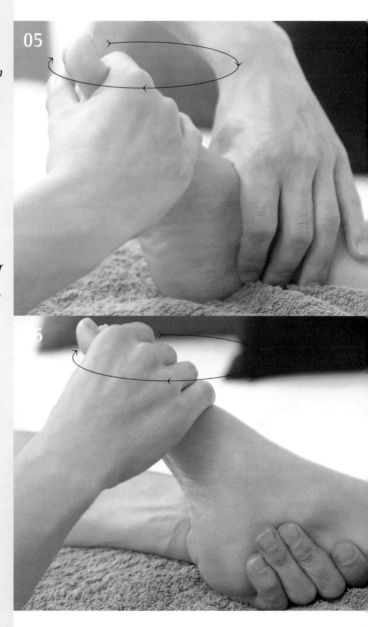

Foot moulding *(07)*
*Holding the top of the foot
between your two palms,
rotate your two hands
around the foot like the
motion of the wheels of a
steam train.*

Rib cage relax *(08)*
*Pressing into the sole of the
foot with your two thumbs,
use the creeping technique
to work across the top of
the foot with the fingers
of both hands.*

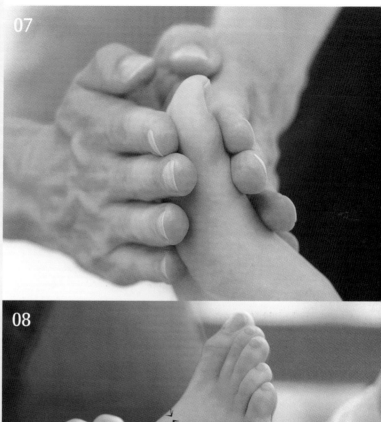

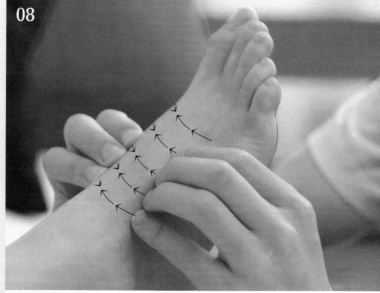

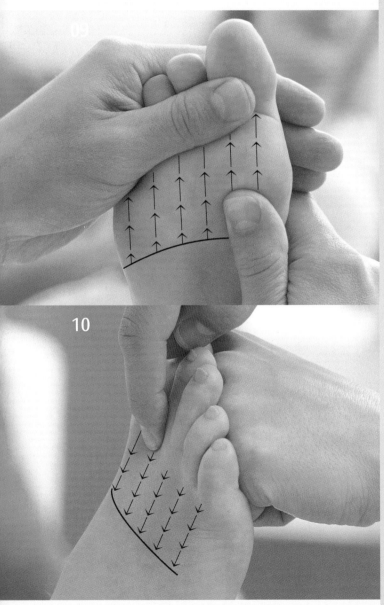

Lung: sole *(09)*
Use the creeping technique to work the area between the diaphragm line and shoulder line on the sole of the foot.

Lung: top of feet *(10)*
Use your index finger to creep down the grooves on top of the foot as shown.

Sinuses *(11)*
For the right foot, hold the top of the foot with your left hand and work with your right thumb; for the left foot, reverse the hand positions.
Starting at the base of the big toe, use the creeping technique to work up all the toes. When you reach the little toe, change hands and work back.

Eye *(12)*
Use the rotating technique to work the eye reflex, which is under the first bend of the second toe. For the right foot, support the top of the foot with the left hand and work the toe with the right; for the left, swap hands.

Ear *(13)*
The ear reflex is located under the first bend of the third toe. As for the eye reflex, work this point using the rotating technique.

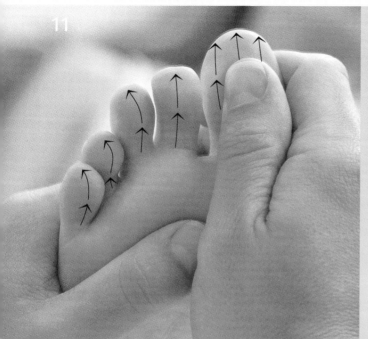

11

SMALLER HEAD POINTS

Reflexes for the pineal gland, pituitary gland, hypothalamus, nose, and throat are located beneath the sinuses on the big toe. You will automatically contact these points when working the sinuses.

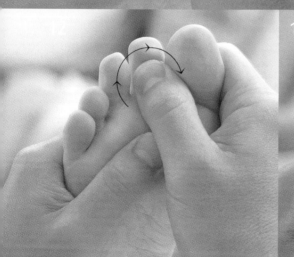

12

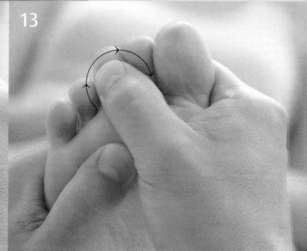

13

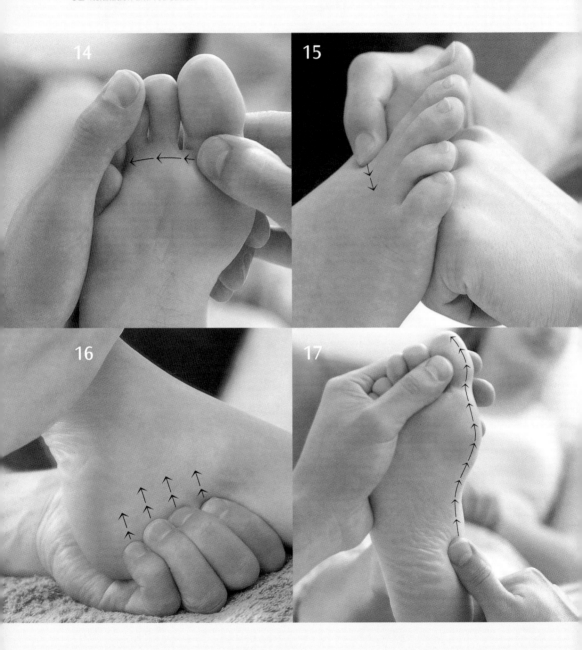

Neck & Thyroid: sole *(14)*
Creep along the base of the first three toes (the shoulder line) three times.

Neck & Thyroid: top *(15)*
Use your index finger to creep three times along the base of the first three toes on top of the foot.

Coccyx, Hip, & Pelvis *(16)*
To work the coccyx on the right foot (16), hold the top of the foot with your right hand. Creep up the inside of the heel with the four fingers of your left hand. For the hip and pelvis, support the right foot with your left hand and use your right to work the outside of the heel. Exchange hands for the left foot.

Spine *(17)*
Creep up the inside edge of the foot to the top of the big toe. Use your right thumb on the right foot and vice versa.

Cervical spine *(18)*
Return to the big toe and use your index finger to creep up the inside edge of the foot.

Chronic neck *(19)*
Work down the outer edge of the first three toes, using your right thumb on the right foot and left thumb on the left.

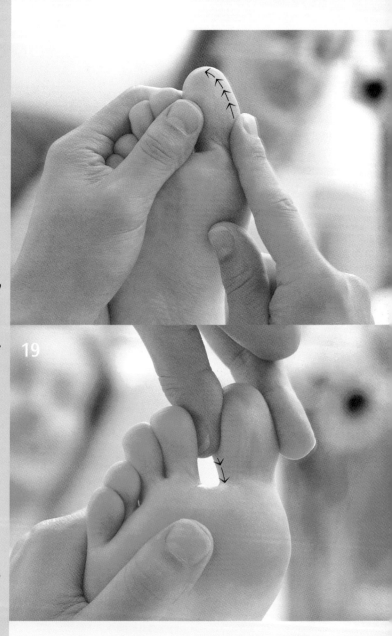

19

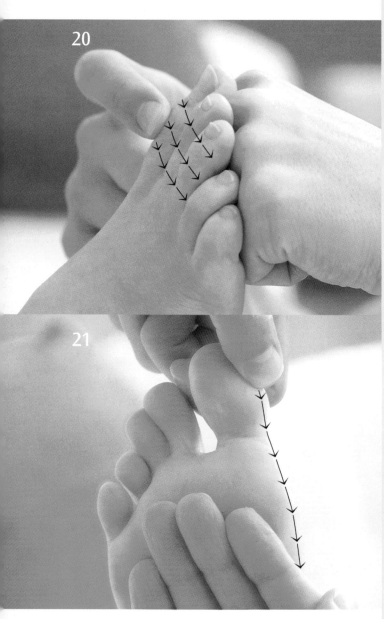

Face (20)
Support the right foot with your left fist. Use your right index finger to creep along the first three toes. Change hands for the left foot.

Spine (Down) (21)
Supporting the sole with the back of your non-working hand, creep down the inside edge of the foot.

Shoulder (22)
Cradling the top of the foot, creep your thumb outwards across the area. Change hands and creep inwards with the other thumb.

Knee & Elbow (23)
Creep your index finger across the triangular-shaped reflex on the outside of the foot.

Primary sciatic (24)
Use your index finger to creep up the area behind the ankle bone, continuing up the leg for about 4cm (1½in).

Secondary sciatic (25)
This area lies across the heel halfway between the pelvic line and bottom of the foot. Creep along this line two or three times from the inside to outside edge of the foot.

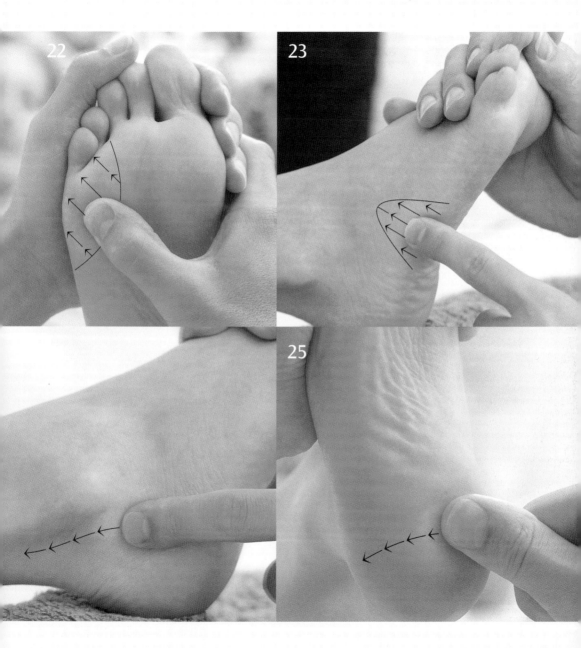

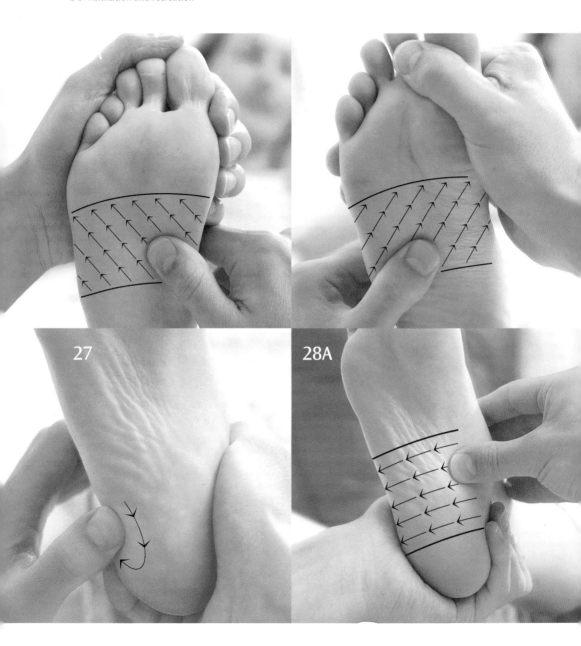

Liver (26, A & B)
This reflex is on the right foot only. Support the foot with your left hand and creep your right thumb across, from the inside to the outside (26A). Change hands and work in the opposite direction (26B).

Ileocecal valve (27)
This reflex is on the right foot only and lies below the pelvic line on the outermost edge of the foot. Work it using the hooking-out technique.

Intestines (28, A & B)
Work the right foot only to contact the ileocecal valve, ascending and transverse colon and small intestines.
  Supporting the heel with your left hand, use your right thumb to work the area under the waist line from the inside to outside (28A). Swap hands and work back (28B).

Urinary system (29)
To contact the bladder and ureter tube, creep up the inside edge of the ligament line to the waist line. The kidney and adrenal lie above where the waist and ligament lines intersect. Use the rotating technique to work this reflex.

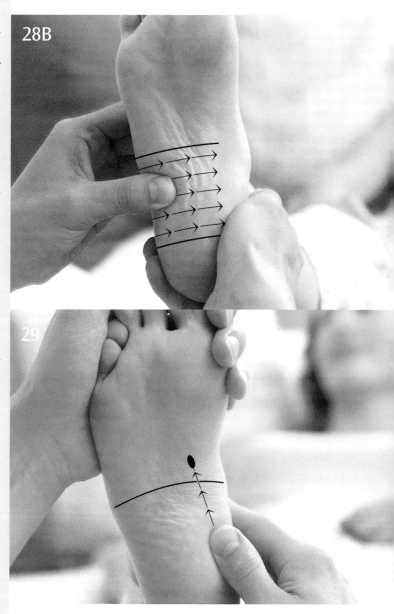

Uterus/Prostate (30)

For the right foot, support it in your left hand and use your right index finger to work from the tip of the heel to the inside ankle bone. The actual reflex point for the uterus/prostrate is midway between the heel and ankle bone. For the left foot, change your supporting hand and work with your left index finger.

Fallopian tube/Vas Deferens (31)

Support the sole of the foot with your two thumbs and, pressing in with them, use your third and index fingers on both hands to creep across the top of the foot. Repeat two or three times.

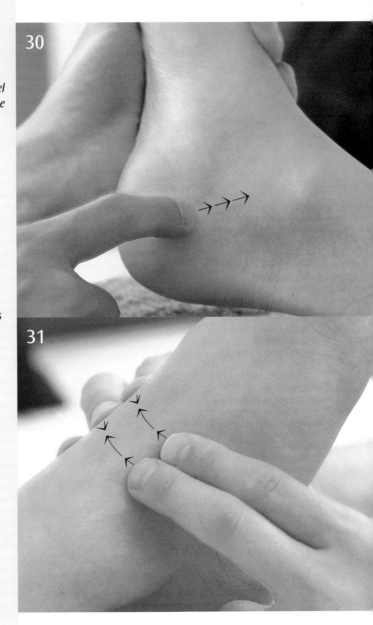

Ovary/Testis *(32)*

This is similar to working the uterus/prostate reflex, only this time you work the outside edge of the foot.

To work the right foot, support it in your left hand and use your right index finger to creep from the tip of the heel to the outside ankle bone. The actual reflex point for the ovary/testis is halfway between the heel and ankle bone. For the left foot, support it with your right hand and work with your left index finger.

Heart *(33)*

The main reflex for the heart is on the left foot only. It is a rectangular-shaped reflex that sits on the diaphragm line beneath the first three toes. It finishes halfway between the diaphragm and shoulder lines. Don't treat this area more than three times, as you will have already worked it when contacting the lung—reflexes overlap like organs do in the body.

Supporting the top of the left foot with your right hand, creep your left thumb across from the big toe to the third toe, then give the diaphragm relaxation exercise on p.86.

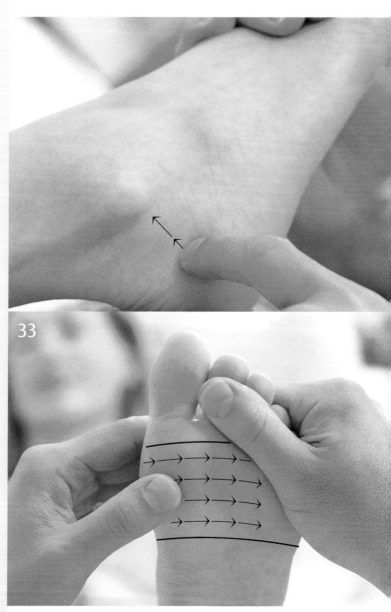

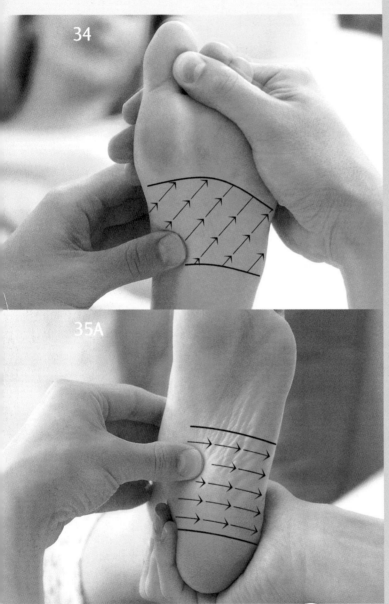

Stomach (34)

The main stomach reflex is on the left foot between the diaphragm and waist lines.

Support the left foot with your right hand. Working from the inside to the outside of the foot, use your left thumb to contact the area shown. Swap hands and work in the opposite direction with your right thumb.

Intestines (35, A & B)

The intestines on the left foot include the small intestines and transverse, descending, and, below the pelvic line (36), sigmoid colon.

Support the heel with your right hand and use your left thumb to work the area under the waist line from the inside to outside edge (35A). Swap hands and work in the opposite direction (35B).

Sigmoid colon (36)

This V-shaped reflex is on the left foot only and is found under the pelvic line.

Hold the base of the heel with your right hand and use your left hand to creep up the outside fork of the V-shaped reflex. Swap hands and work up the inside fork of the V-shape with your right thumb (36).

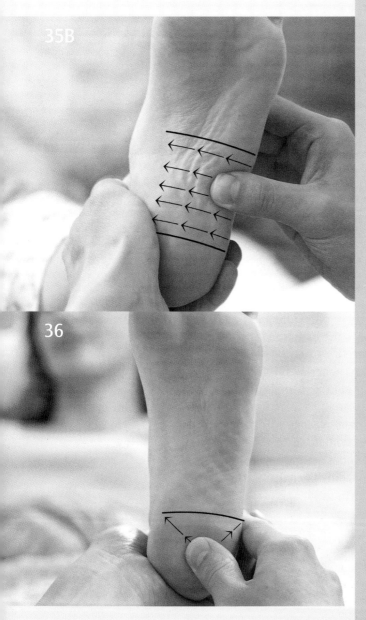

WINDING-DOWN MASSAGE

If certain reflexes are very sensitive, directly massage the corresponding body part. This enhances the treatment and helps the receiver enter a deeper state of relaxation. You don't have to be a massage expert: all you need is a chair or flat surface, your hands, and a little oil. This routine is for the neck, shoulders, and back, which often hold tension.

Step One
Apply a little oil to your palms and use slow, circular movements to massage the receiver's shoulders and up either side of the vertebrae. Use the tips of your index fingers to work up the neck.

Step Two
Starting at the base of the spine, use your palms in circular movements to work up either side of the entire column. Repeat four times.

Step Three
Return to the base of the spine and work up it again, this time making small circular movements with your index fingers. Repeat and then finish by sliding your palms up the spine and out across the shoulders.

Food for a balanced diet

Eating a balanced diet is all-important for our health. We should aim to eat three meals a day: breakfast (see pp.40–1), lunch (see pp.76–7), and a main meal (see pp.104–5), supplemented with a snack if necessary. Most of us know we should eat less meat and fat and more fruit, vegetables, and fibre, yet it is difficult to know if we are achieving the correct balance.

Generally, it is the quality of the food you eat that matters, not the quantity. How much you need depends on your individual height and lifestyle, but as a general rule a meal should fill the equivalent of your cupped hands—any more stresses your digestive system. We need whole, unrefined foods to which nothing has been added or taken away. You must also drink at least 2 litres (3½ pints) of pure, filtered water every day to flush out toxins in the body and keep hydrated. Coffee, tea, and alcohol are particularly dehydrating and age the body, above all the skin. A well-hydrated person has a glowing complexion.

Aim to eat a balance of acid- and alkaline-based foods. Acid-forming foods are meat, eggs, fish, game, starches, and products made from flour. This includes all cereal products. Alkaline foods are high in sodium and potassium. All fruits, including the apparently acidic citric fruits, are alkaline, as well as green and root vegetables, such as cabbage, Brussels sprouts, carrots, and potatoes. Don't peel potatoes, as their skins hold many nutrients. The ideal ratio of acid and alkaline foods in your diet is one to four, so for every portion of cheese, fish, meat, and bread, eat four of fruit and green and root vegetables.

COMMON DEFICIENCIES
Calcium
If your nails break easily, your teeth have cavities, and you feel irritable you may well have a calcium deficiency. Other symptoms include permanently tense neck and shoulder muscles and an oversensitivity to pain. Eat more dark green vegetables, sunflower and sesame seeds, nuts, and oats. Milk is high in calcium, but is not always suitable for people suffering from catarrh and eczema.

Iron
If you always feel tired, lack energy, and have a pallid complexion, you may have anaemia, or an iron deficiency. Women are more likely to become anaemic if they have heavy periods. Molasses are high in iron, as are dark green vegetables and liver.

As a general rule, eat five portions of fresh fruit and vegetables a day and up to four slices of wholemeal bread. Eat fish at least twice a week, poultry once or twice a week, and red meat only once a week. Cheese should only be used in dishes sparingly—grate it rather than slice—while pastry should be reserved for special occasions only. Try to restrict your alcohol intake: one or two glasses to accompany a meal once or twice a week is enough. Use olive oil for cooking rather than ordinary vegetable oil, as it is high in antioxidants and helps lower cholesterol. Avoid eating heavy meals late at night, as it is difficult to sleep soundly when your body is busy digesting.

EATING FOR A BUSY LIFESTYLE

Unfortunately, the first thing that usually suffers when you are extremely busy or stressed is your diet. It is often tempting to eat sugary, quick-fix foods, such as chocolate, during the day as they give the body an instant energy rush, despite leaving you feeling more lethargic when they wear off. For sustained energy, choose instead a banana, a handful of shelled almonds or cashew nuts, some ready-to-eat dried apricots, or a traditional oatcake.

In the evening, many people are simply too tired even to think about cooking at the end of a busy day, so order a takeaway on their way home. Most takeaways and fast foods are high in fat, low in nutrition, and encourage weight gain. However, as you will see on pp.104–5, it takes very little effort to make a healthy and delicious meal in no time at all.

COMMON DEFICIENCIES
Potassium
If you crave salty foods and are having problems sleeping you may be short of potassium. This can lead to water retention, weight gain, and high blood pressure. Reduce your salt intake, eat more bananas, and take kelp supplements. You will soon feel calmer and sleep more soundly.

Vitamin C
If you seem to catch every infection that comes your way, try to eat foods that are high in vitamin C, such as citrus fruits, melon, blackcurrants, berries, red peppers, and broccoli. Vitamin C is excellent for boosting the immune system.

Meals in minutes

It is actually extremely easy to prepare a quick and healthy meal in minutes. All it takes is a little planning at the weekend or beginning of the week and a trip to the supermarket. Many supermarkets cater for the busy person and sell packets of peeled and chopped fresh vegetables, washed lettuces, fresh soups, and fresh sauces. Although you should always check for a high fat or salt content in ready-made soups and sauces, most of these can help you to eat healthily for only a little extra cost. Be inspired by the simple suggestions shown here for quick, healthy, yet extremely tasty options.

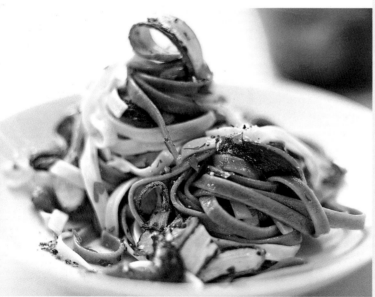

MAIN COURSE

Pasta is an extremely versatile food and can be ready in a few minutes. Brush slices of peppers and courgettes with olive oil and roast while you are waiting for your pasta to cook (spinach and egg tagliatelle shown here). Season with black pepper and garnish with fresh basil.

Alternatively, bake a piece of haddock wrapped in foil together with slices of lime and garlic and sprigs of fresh thyme. Serve with a variety of lightly steamed vegetables, such as baby fennel, carrot, and courgettes, shown here.

DESSERT

Grilled fresh fruit is an excellent way to finish any meal. Sprinkle a little sugar over a mixture of figs, white peaches, and pineapple chunks and place under a hot grill until the sugar starts to caramelize. Try this with any of your favourite fruits.

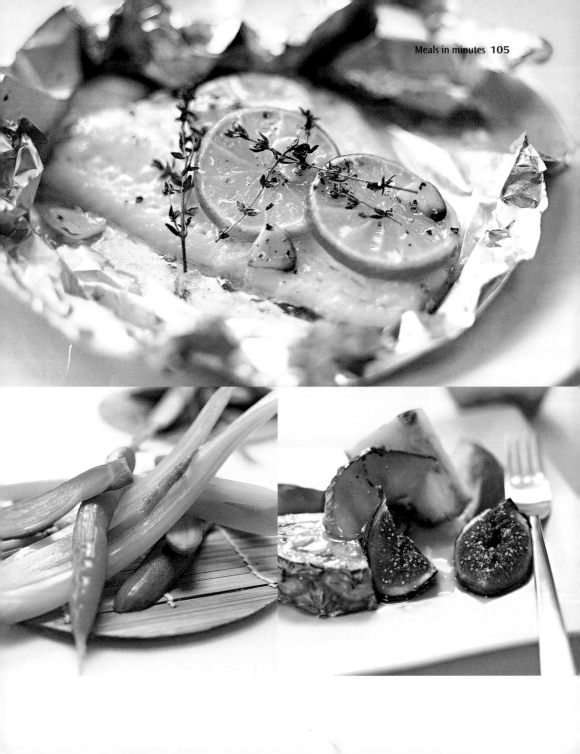

Preparing for sleep

Sound sleep is something we all need but don't always get: an incredible 50 per cent of us have trouble sleeping at some time or other. Caught up in our busy lives, most of us disrupt or ignore our natural body clocks. (To overcome jet lag, see p.59.)

Just as you follow a particular ritual when you arrive home from work, try to establish a routine before you go to bed, signalling to your body that it is time to sleep. A warm aromatherapy bath with a few drops of lavender will encourage sleepiness, otherwise simply wash your face and feet in warm water. Afterwards, spend a few minutes pampering yourself.

If you do not have time for a full reflexology treatment early in the evening, ask your partner or a friend to spend a few minutes relaxing your feet before you go to bed. (This is more relaxing than treating your own hands.) Simply follow the diaphragm and metatarsal relaxation exercises on pp.86–7.

INSOMNIA

If you suffer from insomnia you will know that the more you try to sleep the harder it becomes. Often the best thing to do is to sit up with a hot drink and a soporific book. General worries about relationships, work, health, and finances can keep you awake at night, although persistent insomnia is often linked to a deeper anxiety about life, and depression. If sleeping problems persist, ask yourself what you can do to ease your worries and improve your lifestyle, and consider seeking professional advice. Avoid prescription sleeping pills, as these are addictive and cause further

YOUR BEDROOM
Ensure your bedroom is an inviting and calming space to sleep in. Keep it as clutter-free and clean as possible and sleep with the window open to improve air quality unless it is very noisy or humid outside. An ionizer will also improve the atmosphere.

problems; instead, try taking valerian either as a tea or as a tincture. Alternatively, prepare an infusion of chamomile or limeflowers. All of these will help you relax and promote good sleep.

GENERAL SELF-HELP

■ Don't consume any caffeine after 7pm or cut it out of your diet altogether. Dandelion coffee and herbal teas, such as chamomile, are good substitutes for tea and coffee.
■ Ensure that your diet is properly balanced (see pp.102–3) and make a habit of not eating any later than 8pm. Avoid high protein foods, such as cheese, steak, or beef burgers, as you will not sleep peacefully if your stomach is digesting a heavy meal.
■ Try taking a calcium and magnesium supplement before you go to bed.
■ It is vital that you are comfortable in bed. Your bed should be firm yet allow your spine to rest in its natural S-shape when you lie flat. An unsuitable bed will cause back pain and sleepless nights.
■ Make sure you are not too hot or too cold and adjust the bedclothes accordingly.
■ Sprinkle a few drops of chamomile or lavender essential oils on to a tissue and place it on your pillow.
■ Try drinking a glass of warmed milk with 1 tsp of honey and a pinch of cinnamon. (Avoid milk if you have catarrh or eczema.)
■ Breathing slowly and deeply helps sleeplessness. Lie with your hand on your diaphragm and concentrate on its rising and falling with each in- and out-breath.

MELATONIN PRODUCTION
Melatonin (see also p.59) occurs naturally in the body—the pineal gland secretes it mainly at night—and helps it prepare for sleep by lowering the heart rate and reducing alertness. If street lighting is able to shine in to your bedroom it may lower your melatonin levels and thereby discourage sleep. Invest in thick curtains or adjust the position of your bed.

However, you should also guard against having too much melatonin in your body, as this can make you feel depressed. As a general rule, you can balance the body's natural production of melatonin with a healthy diet and exercise. Try also to take brisk walks in the morning sunshine or, during dark winter days, to sit under bright artificial light.

CHAPTER SIX

Prevention
& cure

Because reflexology is most effective when
applied to the feet, try to follow up a hand
treatment with a foot treatment when you get
home. This section focuses on the feet and
which reflexes you should work to overcome
and prevent common conditions.

For longer-term or more serious conditions it is advisable to complement your sessions at home with regular visits to a qualified reflexology practitioner (see Resources for details of how to find one). Equally, if you are in any doubt about a condition, you must seek professional advice.

To treat one of the conditions in this section, follow the entire reflexology foot routine on pp.86–101 and then spend a few extra minutes on the individual reflexes shown. If time is at a premium you can just work the relevant reflexes for a given ailment after warming up the foot with the relaxation exercises on pp.86–9. Always complete the entire sequence on the right foot before repeating the treatment on the left foot.

Preventing illness is just as important as curing illness, and as a general rule a healthy person should aim to receive a full reflexology foot treatment at least once a month (see also p.35). If you are healthy but susceptible to a condition, your monthly treatment should concentrate on the appropriate reflexes.

It is also important to look after your body in between reflexology sessions, as many problems are caused by unhealthy lifestyles and eating habits. The general self-help sections offer advice for individual illnesses, although you should also refer back to the pages on diet, sleeping, travelling, etc. If you look after yourself, body and mind, you will not only enjoy long-term good health but also feel happier and more relaxed.

Allergies & asthma

An allergy is a physical reaction to one or more allergens or irritants, for example pollen, certain foods, such as wheat or dairy products, food additives, detergents, or animal fur. Stress can also trigger allergies as it weakens immunity. Asthma is often an allergic reaction, although it has been linked to poor air quality in inner cites. Other common allergic symptoms include rashes, hay fever, and migraine. When treating an allergy, rather than focusing on the reaction, try to discover why the body is allergic.

Reflexology works by reducing stress levels and strengthening the body, in particular the digestive and immune systems. After relaxing the feet (see pp.86–9), work the feet as shown right. For self-help, work the entire area of the palms of both hands to contact the reflexes for the digestive and respiratory systems.

GENERAL SELF-HELP

■ Eat a balanced diet (see pp.102–3) and try to eliminate all refined sugars and additives, particularly orange and yellow food dyes and monosodium glutamate.
■ Take vitamin C supplements in the morning before eating or drinking. Cut down on tea, coffee, and salt.
■ Keep your house clean and dust free and don't use artificial air fresheners.
■ Drink thyme or lavender herbal tea, both of which have an antiseptic action and help break down mucus.
■ Practise deep breathing regularly (see p.37) and exercise your respiratory system. Swimming is ideal if you are susceptible to pollen or dust.

REFLEXOLOGY
Lung: sole *(01)*
Use the creeping technique to work the area between the diaphragm line and shoulder line on the sole of the foot.

Intestines *(02)*
For the right foot, support the heel with your left hand and use your right thumb to work the area under the waist line from the inside to outside. Swap hands and work back. For the left foot, reverse all hand positions.

Liver *(03)*
This reflex is on the right foot only. Support the foot with your left hand and creep your right thumb across, from the inside to the outside. Change hands and work back in the opposite direction.

Stomach *(04)*
Support the left foot with your right hand. Working from the inside to the outside of the foot, use your left thumb to contact the area shown. Swap hands and use your right thumb to work in the opposite direction.

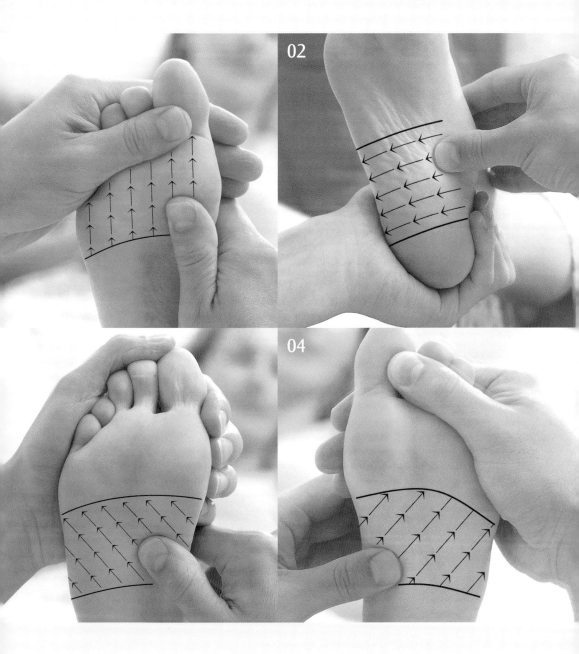

Conjunctivitis

Poor lighting, artificial lighting, a smoky atmosphere, staring at a screen for long periods of time, and emotional stresses and strains all take their toll on your eyesight (see also p.73). However, conjunctivitis is usually caused by a localized infection in the sinuses, which spreads into the delicate mucous membranes of the eyes. The eyes feel painful and itchy, the whites of the eyes become slightly pink, and the inside edge of each eye emits an unpleasant, yellow, sticky discharge.

When working with reflexology for conjunctivitis or indeed any eye condition, work out the entire head and sinus area, as well as the actual eye reflex. For self-help, work the sinus and eye reflexes on both hands.

GENERAL SELF-HELP
■ *Use eye drops and bathe your eyes frequently in a mild solution of salt water.*
■ *Relax with a witch hazel cold compress twice daily. Soak cotton wool pads in diluted witch hazel. Chill them in the fridge for 15 minutes and then relax in a comfortable chair with the pads on your eyes. This also soothes tired, sore eyes, reduces puffiness, and helps you generally unwind.*

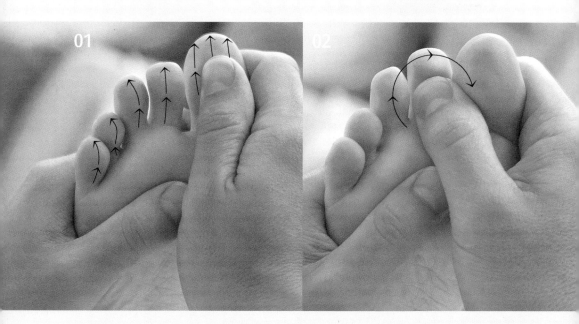

REFLEXOLOGY

Sinuses (01)
For the right foot, hold the top of the foot with your left hand; for the left, change hands. Starting at the base of the big toe, use the creeping technique to work up all the toes. When you reach the little toe, change hands and work back.

Eye (02)
Use the rotating technique to contact the eye reflex, which is located below the first bend of the second toe. For the right foot, support the top of the foot with the left hand and work the toe with the right. Swap hands when treating the left foot.

Face (03)
Support the sole of the right foot with the fist of your left hand. Use your right index finger to creep along the first three toes. Change hands for the left foot .

HEALTHY EATING, HEALTHY EYES

A good diet is essential for healthy eyes. Eat more legumes, which are high in sulphur and therefore amino acids, yellow vegetables, which contain carotenes, rich berries (blackberries, bilberries, and cherries), which contain flavonoids, and all foods with high levels of vitamin C (kiwi fruits and strawberries).

For tired, strained eyes take ginkgo biloba supplements, which will also help macular degeneration. Other supplements you might consider taking are vitamins C and E, zinc, and selenium, all of which will boost your nutritional intake and therefore the health of your eyes.

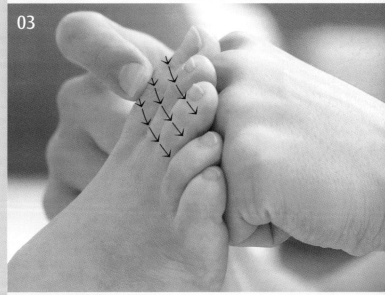

03

Cystitis

Cystitis is an inflammatory bladder condition that is common in women, as the bladder, uterus, and rectum are in close proximity to each other and the urethra is short. Symptoms include a burning sensation on passing urine, a desire to urinate frequently, discomfort in the lower pelvic region, and feeling generally unwell.

The causes are many: wearing tight-fitting trousers, as this restricts circulation to the vaginal area and creates a moist, bacteria-friendly environment; not drinking enough fluids so urine stagnates; taking antibiotics for a localized infection, as this can affect your immune system; bruising the vaginal and bladder

GENERAL SELF-HELP
- Drink plenty of spring water throughout the day.
- Apple cider vinegar is a great antiseptic. Take 2 tsps in a large tumbler of warm water twice a day.
- Take 1 tsp of bicarbonate of soda and the juice of half a fresh lemon in a glass of warm water.
- Massage a little tea tree oil into your abdomen, working with circular strokes as low down as your pubic line.

REFLEXOLOGY
Urinary system (01)
For the right foot, support the top of the foot with your left hand and work with your right thumb. Reverse hands for the left foot.

To contact the bladder and ureter tube creep up the inside edge of the ligament line to the waist line. Don't work on the ligament itself.

The kidney lies above the point where the waist and ligament lines intersect. Use the rotating technique to contact this reflex.

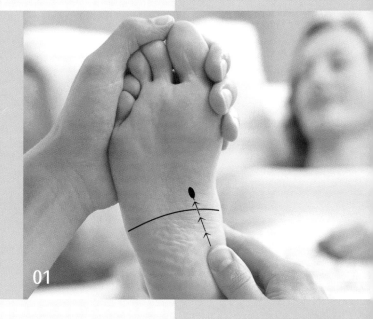

01

walls during intercourse. Taking the birth control pill also lowers immunity, probably because it affects vitamin C stores in the body, and is the second most common cause of cystitis.

Reflexology can greatly relieve cystitis, especially when the feet are worked. Concentrate on the reflexes for the urinary system, namely the bladder, ureter tubes, and kidneys. You should also work the spine to improve the nerve and blood supply to the pelvic region. The most important area of the spine to work is the lumbar spine, which is between the pelvic and waist lines. If you are unable to treat the feet, work the urinary system and the spine reflexes on the hands.

CAUTION
If symptoms are very painful and distressing or persist after 48 hours, seek medical advice.

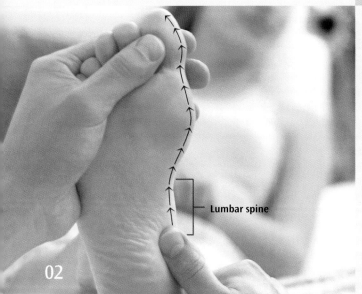

Lumbar spine

02

Spine *(02)*
Support the feet in the same way as you did when working the urinary system.

To contact the spine, creep your working thumb up the inside edge of the foot, from the base of the heel to the top of the big toe. Return to the part of the spine reflex between the pelvic and waist lines and work over this area again. This contacts the lumbar spine, the five vertebrae between the bottom of the ribs and the hip bones.

Depression & addictions

Everybody has days or periods in their lives when they feel sad, depressed, or worried, often in response to a particular event. Classic symptoms vary from anxiety, mood swings, and insomnia to fatigue, loss of appetite and concentration, and general apathy.

Depression and addictions are often related as people typically turn to comforting substances when they are depressed. Some addictions are relatively harmless or considered socially acceptable while others seriously damage your health. Being patient and allowing yourself time to recover is often the best remedy for depression, although there are also many other options that offer great comfort. For example,

GENERAL SELF-HELP
- *Eat a balanced diet (see pp.102–3) and sleep for at least eight hours every night.*
- *Take plenty of exercise to release endorphins, the body's natural analgesic.*
- *Take St John's wort, a non-addictive antidepressant, in capsule form or as a tea.*
- *Regular aromatherapy massages using rose, neroli, frankincense, or bergamot are particularly good for counteracting depression.*

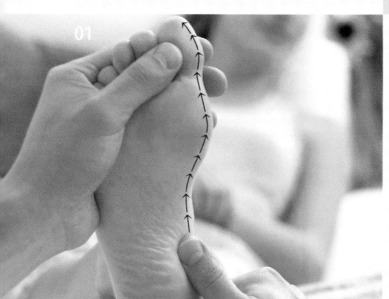

REFLEXOLOGY

Spine (01)
Creep up the inside edge of the foot to the top of the big toe. Use the right hand on the right foot and vice versa.

Cervical spine (02)
Return to the big toe and use your index finger to creep up the outside edge of it in a finer movement.

Spine (Down) (03)
Supporting the sole with the back of your non-working hand, creep down the inside edge of the foot.

sharing your worries, either with friends and family or a professional counsellor, helps counteract feelings of isolation or loneliness. There are also many support networks that will help you overcome addictions, such as smoking, alcoholism, and drugs. Consult your doctor or local directory for details.

The healing touch of reflexology can bring great comfort, both physically and emotionally. It will also help heal any physical imbalance in the body. Concentrate on the central nervous system, spine, and brain reflexes. It is possible to work your own hands during low points in the day. Concentrate on the spine and brain reflexes.

ANTIDEPRESSANTS

If you do decide to take antidepressants, be very careful to increase your intake of fresh fruit and vegetables as well as oily fish. This is because antidepressants tend to deplete essential nutrients in the body, particularly amino acids, which can affect the normal functioning of the brain and add to your depression.

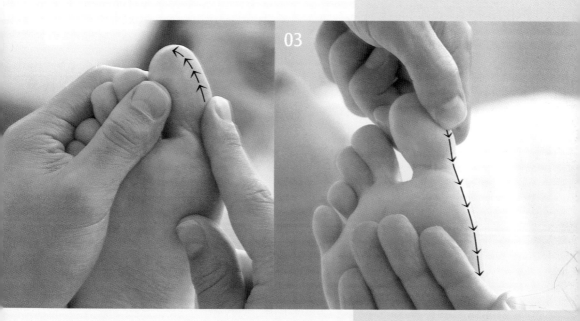

03

Earache & sinusitis

When adults suffer from earache it is often as a result of a heavy head cold or an acute attack of sinusitis. Ear infections usually affect the middle ear and are extremely painful. For acute earache always seek immediate medical attention, as the infection can easily be carried to the brain.

The sinuses are bony, porous, hollow cavities in the facial area, which resemble the texture of a teabag. The sinuses give resonance to the voice, act as filters for mucus, and lighten the weight of the head on the neck. Sinusitis is an extremely painful inflammation of the sinuses, where the porous cavities swell and get blocked with sticky mucus. It is also common to lose the sense of taste and smell. If left untreated, the infection often spreads to the ears and causes earache.

GENERAL SELF-HELP
Your doctor will probably recommend antibiotics. Try also the suggestions below.
■ *Rest in bed if you have an acute attack of sinusitis. Drink plenty of fluids, such as diluted vegetable juices, soups, and herbal teas.*
■ *Remove from your diet all refined sugars and mucus-forming foods.*
■ *For sinusitis, try resting with a hot flannel on your face; for earache, place a well-wrapped hot water bottle on the affected ear.*

REFLEXOLOGY

Sinuses (01)
For the right foot, hold the top of the foot with your left hand; for the left, reverse the hand positions. Starting at the base of the big toe, use the creeping technique to work up all the toes. When you reach the little toe, change hands and work back.

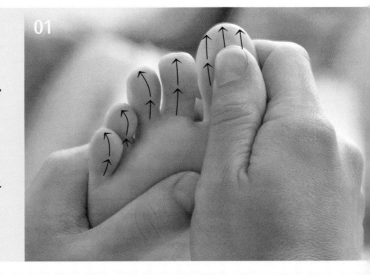
01

Acute bacterial sinusitis is commonly caused by a head cold, hay fever, or even a dental infection, while chronic sinus infections are usually linked to an allergy or sensitivity to a household chemical, such as an air freshener, perfume, or hair spray.

Reflexology will help to provide relief from the pain of sinusitis and earache and assist the body in fighting off the infection. When treating sinusitis it is essential that you work both the ear and the sinus reflexes to discourage the infection from spreading to the ear. For self-help, treat the equivalent reflexes on the hands, namely the sinus and ear.

GENERAL SELF-HELP
■ *Prepare a wintergreen or juniper inhalation (see p.42) to help congested sinuses clear and ease pain.*
■ *Take 10 drops of echinacea tincture, a herbal immune stimulant, up to three times daily during the infection and then once daily for a complete month when it has cleared. This is particularly important if you have been taking antibiotics.*

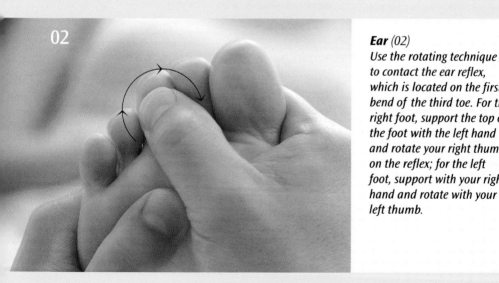

02

Ear (02)
Use the rotating technique to contact the ear reflex, which is located on the first bend of the third toe. For the right foot, support the top of the foot with the left hand and rotate your right thumb on the reflex; for the left foot, support with your right hand and rotate with your left thumb.

Fertility

If a woman is between 22 and 30 years old and wanting to conceive, she can expect to try for about nine months. Fertility is closely linked to lifestyle and diet, so both partners must take steps to deal with everyday stress and eat a balanced diet. A woman is at her most fertile between the 12th and 16th days of her cycle, so keep a diary to pinpoint this period. (The first day of menstruation is considered day one of a woman's cycle.) If you are concerned about your or your partner's fertility arrange for a fertility test.

Reflexology improves hormonal function, reduces stress, and encourages conception. Take it in turns at home to treat each other two or three times a week. For best results you may also need to enlist the help of a professional and follow a treatment for three or four months. Work the central nervous system and brain as well as the entire endocrine system, namely the pituitary, pineal, thyroid, and adrenal glands as well as the ovaries/testes. You should also contact the hypothalamus, which coordinates the endocrine and nervous systems and is involved in motivating sexual behaviour. The hypothalamus is located behind the eyes in the brain and is about the size of a pea. For self-help, work the reflexes for the spine, brain, adrenals, endocrine system, and the ovaries/testes.

GENERAL SELF-HELP FOR BOTH PARTNERS
- Give up smoking, cut out alcohol and all food additives, and reduce caffeine intake.
- Take ginseng and zinc supplements.
- Take plenty of gentle exercise, such as yoga or tai chi.

REFLEXOLOGY
Spine & Brain *(01)*
Creep up the inside edge of the foot to the top of the big toe. Use the right hand on the right foot and vice versa.

Neck & Thyroid: sole *(02)*
Creep along the base of the first three toes three times.

Neck & Thyroid: top *(03)*
On top of the foot, creep your index finger three times along the base of the first three toes .

Ovary/Testis *(04)*
Use your index finger to creep from the tip of the heel to the outside ankle bone.

Adrenal *(05)*
The adrenal reflex is on top of the kidney reflex on the inside of the ligament line. Use a deep rotation to contact this reflex.

Pituitary, Pineal, & Hypothalamus *(06)*
Supporting the top of the foot, creep your thumb up the big toe three times. Work only from the outside of the big toe to the middle.

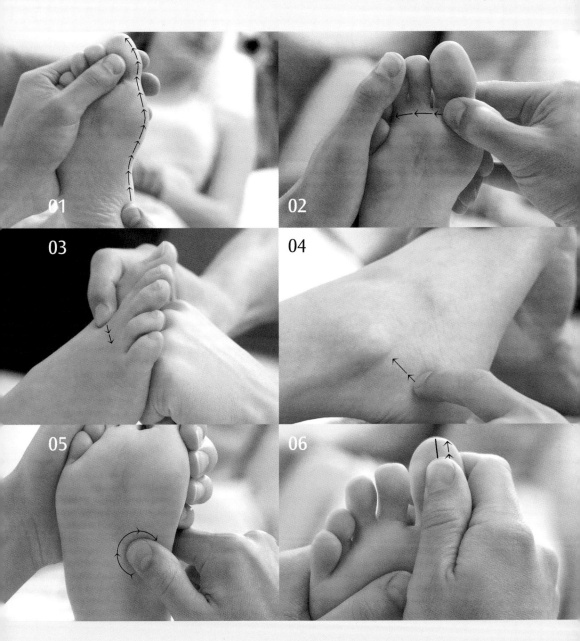

Headaches & migraine

Most headaches (see also pp.44–5) clear quite rapidly within a day and are usually caused by eye strain, too much rich food and drink the previous day, stress, or a bacterial or viral infection.

Migraine (see also pp.74–5) is a surprisingly common disorder affecting 15 to 20 per cent of men and 25 to 30 per cent of women. Classical symptoms include severe throbbing pain on one or both sides of the head, nausea, blurring or bright spots in the vision, anxiety, fatigue, and sometimes tingling of the arms and legs.

Reflexology will quickly relieve a headache or migraine, particularly if the feet are treated. For a migraine work the liver, cervical spine, neck, and thyroid. Omit the liver when treating a headache.

REFLEXOLOGY
Liver (01)
This reflex is on the right foot only and should be worked when treating a migraine.

Support the foot with your left hand and creep your right thumb across, from the inside to the outside. Change hands and work in the opposite direction.

Cervical spine (02)
For the right foot, hold the top of the foot with your left hand and creep your right index finger up the outside edge of the big toe. Repeat two or three times. Change hands for the left foot.

Neck & Thyroid: sole (03)
Creep along the base of the first three toes three times. For the right foot support with your left and work with your right thumb. Swap hands for the left foot.

Neck & Thyroid: top (04)
For the right foot, support the foot with your left fist. Creep your index finger three times along the base of the first three toes. Reverse hand positions for the left foot.

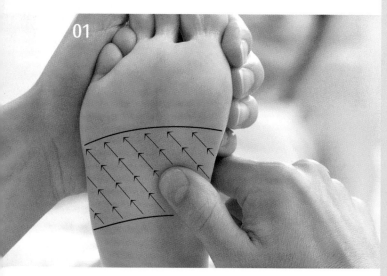

01

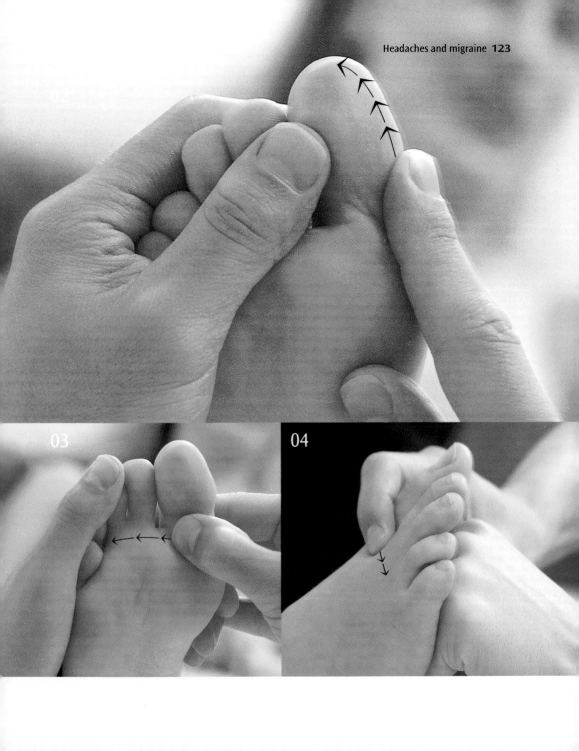

High blood pressure

Hypertension or high blood pressure is one of the major medical problems in the West and is associated with cardiovascular illness. This is because the increased pressure of blood flowing through the delicate nephrons in the kidneys stresses the renal system and in turn the cardiovascular system. Bad diet, including drinking too much alcohol and caffeine, is most closely related to hypertension, although a general lack of exercise and inability to cope with emotional stress compound the problem.

Reflexology lowers blood pressure by treating the renal system, namely the bladder, ureter, and kidneys. This is a condition that requires longer-term, regular treatment, so keep persisting.

HIGH RISK GROUPS
People who smoke, are overweight or diabetic, or have elevated blood cholesterol levels are most at risk from developing high blood pressure. It is also more common in men.

If you fall into any of these categories you must take steps to safeguard your health. Give up smoking, lose weight, eat healthily, and take regular exercise. If you are very unfit, ask your doctor for a suitable fitness regime.

REFLEXOLOGY
Bladder & Ureter (01)
Creep up the inside edge of the ligament line to the waist line. However, it is important not to work on the ligament line itself as it is very sensitive.

For the right foot, support the top of the foot with your left hand and work with your right thumb. Reverse hands for the left foot.

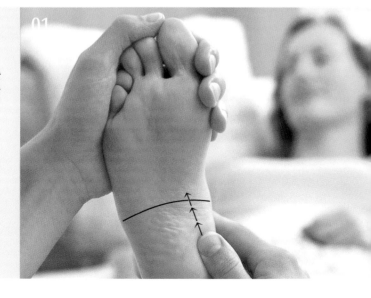

GENERAL SELF-HELP
■ A healthy, balanced diet (see pp.102–3) is essential. Eat more fibre and less salt. Too much salt ultimately stresses the kidneys.
■ Cut out or reduce your intake of alcohol and caffeine.
■ If you find yourself getting stressed during the day, practise deep breathing (see p.37).
■ Learn how to relax properly and make sure you unwind at the end of every day. Relaxation techniques such as biofeedback, autogenics, transcendental meditation, yoga, and hypnosis all reduce stress, which in turn will lower your blood pressure. Experiment with different methods until you find one that suits you.

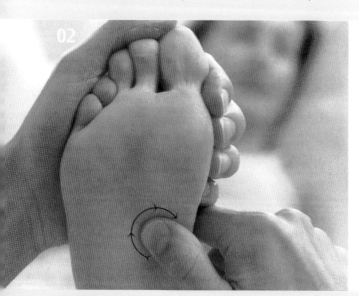

Kidney (02)
The kidney reflex lies above the point where the waist and ligament lines intersect. To work this reflex use a deep rotation with your thumb.

For the right foot, support with your left hand and work with your right thumb. For the left foot, support with your right hand and work with your left thumb.

Indigestion

Indigestion is caused by a combination of dietary- and stress-related factors. For this reason, don't eat when you are upset or angry and instead wait until you feel calm. Always chew your food thoroughly and don't eat "on the run". In the evenings, try to eat before 8pm and avoid heavy foods or large meals. Eating late at night can prevent you from sleeping. You should also ensure that your mealtime is restful. Sit at a table and turn off any loud background music. Resist watching television, above all aggressive or violent programmes. It is not only what you eat but also how you eat that is important.

Reflexology will quickly ease indigestion. Work out the reflexes for the entire digestive system. On the right foot you will find reflexes for the liver, gall bladder, ileocecal valve, ascending and transverse colon, and small intestines. On the left foot you will contact the stomach, pancreas, transverse, descending, and sigmoid colon, as well as the small intestines. For self-help, work both palms (see pp.80–1) to contact the equivalent digestive reflexes.

GENERAL SELF-HELP

■ If you suffer from regular indigestion, keep a food diary to try and pinpoint culprit foods. Rich, fatty, or spicy foods and onions are common culprits.
■ Don't eat too much or you will stress your digestive system—the equivalent of what you can hold in your cupped hands is sufficient.
■ For remedies, see pp.80–1.

REFLEXOLOGY
Liver & Gall Bladder (01)
Support the right foot only with your left hand and creep your right thumb across, from the inside to outside. Change hands and work back.

Stomach & Pancreas (02)
Support the left foot only with your right hand. Creep your left thumb across the foot as shown. Swap hands and work back again.

Intestines (03–04)
Support the right heel (03) with your left hand. Creep your right thumb across the area as shown. Change hands and work back (04). Reverse hands for the left foot.

Ileocecal valve (05)
Work this reflex on the outer edge of the right foot only, hooking out.

Sigmoid colon (06)
Hold the base of the heel with your right hand and use your left thumb to creep up the outside fork of the "V". Swap hands and work up the inside fork with your right thumb.

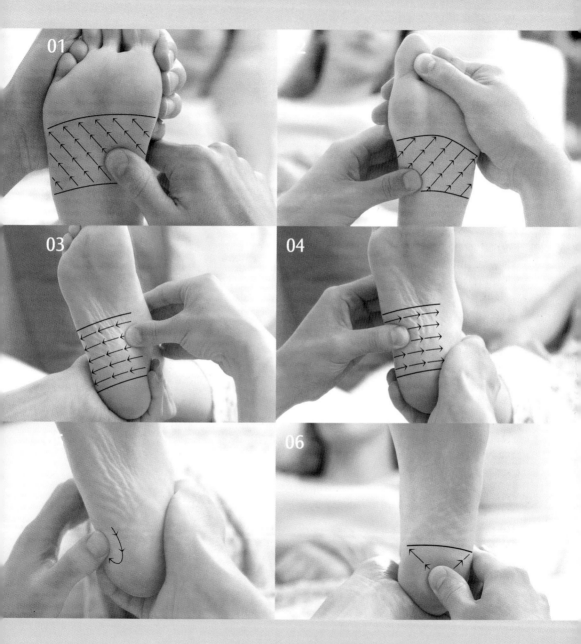

Influenza & colds

Although double-glazing, central heating, fitted carpets, and air conditioning certainly make our lives more comfortable, they also create the perfect conditions for viruses and bacteria to multiply in their millions.

For a cold (see also pp.42–3), the best thing you can do is to let it run its course and make yourself as comfortable as possible. Unless you have a temperature, you can use reflexology to treat certain symptoms of a cold, such as a headache (see pp.44–5 and pp.122–3), earache or sinusitis (see pp.118–19), and throat infections (see pp.136–7). You must also drink plenty of liquids, as it is very easy to become dehydrated with a runny nose.

An attack of influenza, or flu, can make you feel really dreadful and can be quite serious, although it will normally subside within a week. Symptoms include a high temperature, painful aching limbs, a severe headache, and total bodily weakness. Do not be discouraged if you lose your appetite, as this allows your body to focus on fighting the viruses and bacteria. Unless there are associated complications, such as a chest infection, again it is best simply to rest in bed and drink plenty of fluids. If you are very uncomfortable, take painkillers to relieve the symptoms and control your fever.

When you have a raised temperature it will feel very uncomfortable if somebody works the reflexes on your feet or if you work your own hands. For this reason, the relaxation exercises on pp.86–9 for the feet and p.38 for the hands are the only recommended reflexology treatment. You will find these exercises

GENERAL SELF-HELP
At the very first signs of infection, take the following steps to try and prevent your symptoms from developing into a full-blown attack of flu.
■ *Drink plenty of fluids, especially spring water.*
■ *Take echinacea in tincture form three times a day to boost your immune system.*
■ *Take a reasonably hot bath, dispersing six drops of tea tree oil in the water before you get in. Afterwards, retire to bed. Repeat this for the next two or three days.*
■ *If you already feel too ill to bathe, take a tea tree inhalation three times a day. Add five drops of tea tree essential oil to a bowl of hot water. Place a towel over your head and lean over the bowl, breathing slowly and deeply.*

very comforting, particularly if your partner or a friend treats your feet. They will also help alleviate bodily aches and pains.

DETOXING AFTER FLU OR A HEAVY COLD

Often you will feel lacking in energy and generally under the weather after flu or a heavy cold, in which case you should give yourself a detox boost. The Grape Cure is a very effective cleansing diet and is also safe and gentle. For best results follow it for at least three days, for example over a weekend when you are not busy. For the first couple of days you may feel tired or develop a headache, which are positive signs of the body detoxifying. On the third day you should begin to feel more energized. When breaking your fast, do it slowly. Start by eating a little vegetable soup or some salad with fish. The following day add some brown rice with tofu or a little chicken. Gradually return to a normal eating pattern.

GRAPE DETOX PLAN

This detox plan is very simple. Eat four or five meals of grapes each day. (A meal is the amount of grapes you can hold in your two cupped hands.) Use red or white grapes but do not buy the seedless varieties: you need to consume the skin and pips, as there is a substance in the seeds that stimulates the bowel. Chew the pips thoroughly until they resemble grains of sand. Drink at least 4 litres (7 pints) of pure mineral water each day to wash away the toxins that the grapes release from your system.

Irritable bowel syndrome

Irritable bowel syndrome (IBS) is a common condition affecting the function of the large intestine or colon. Sometimes known as spastic colitis, mucus colitis, or intestinal neurosis, IBS generally affects high-striving perfectionists who have great difficulty relaxing. Characteristic symptoms include abdominal pain and distension, more frequent bowel movements, constipation, diarrhoea, flatulence, nausea, anorexia, and varying degrees of anxiety, depression, fatigue, and hostile feelings. See pp.82–3 for causes and detailed general self-help.

For accute irritable bowel syndrome you should aim to receive at least three reflexology foot treatments a week, as well as enlist the help of a practitioner. You should also intersperse foot treatments with regular

IBS FACTS

■ *It is thought that up to 15 per cent of adults suffer from IBS at some point in their lives.*
■ *IBS is more common in women than men.*
■ *Food intolerance and mental distress are the main causes of IBS.*
■ *People with IBS neither lose weight nor become malnourished.*

REFLEXOLOGY

Intestines *(01)*
The intestines on the right foot include the transverse and ascending colon, as well as the small intestine and ileocecal valve.

Supporting the heel with your left hand, use your right thumb to work the area under the waist line from the inside to the outside. Swap hands and work back.

01

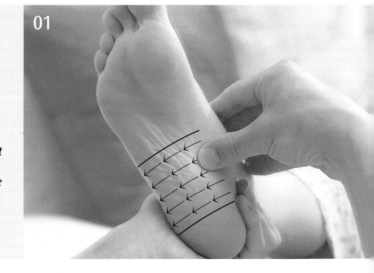

self-help hand treatments (see pp.82–3), particularly after eating. When working either the hands or the feet, concentrate on the intestinal reflexes.

GENERAL SELF-HELP
■ Take a good look at your lifestyle and consider psychotherapy in the form of biofeedback training or hypnotherapy, which will help you learn how to control your anxiety. Mental stress often affects the digestive system, so if you deal with your mental distress your IBS symptoms may well disappear.
■ Increase the amount of physical exercise you take. Exercise helps release tension held in the body and in turn relaxes the bowel.

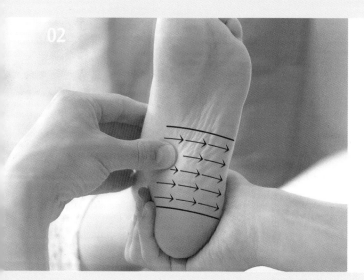

02

Intestines (02)
The intestines on the left foot include the small intestine and transverse, descending, and sigmoid colon.
  Support the heel with your right hand and use your left thumb to work the area under the waist line from the inside to outside edge. Swap hands and work in the opposite direction.

Panic attacks

Over-anxiety, stress, and depression are commonly behind panic attacks. For information on symptoms and how to use reflexology to deal with an attack see pp.52–3. For longer-term treatment ask a friend or loved one to give you regular reflexology foot treatments and body massages at home to help you learn how to relax. As well as the physical benefits—reflexology helps balance the body and mind and will generally help you release any tension—the intimacy between giver and receiver helps heal feelings of isolation and self-doubt.

Your treatment will be much more effective if you have the time to follow the complete foot treatment on pp.86–101 and then spend a few extra minutes working the lungs. The diaphragm relaxation exercise is the most important of the warming-up exercises and you should repeat it four or five times on each foot.

LONG-TERM SELF-HELP
Take a good look at your lifestyle if you suffer from regular panic attacks, particularly if you have low self-esteem or feel depressed.
- Eat a balanced diet (see pp.102–3) and cut out all stimulants, such as caffeine, alcohol, and nicotine.
- Take regular exercise to burn off nervous energy. Swimming, cycling, and vigorous walking are ideal.
- Learn to relax properly. The relaxation exercise on p.85 is a simple yet effective meditation technique for finding serenity in a busy or stressful day.
- Don't be afraid to seek help or advice from others.

REFLEXOLOGY
Diaphragm relax (01)
For the right foot, support the top of the foot with your left hand and use your right thumb to work along the diaphragm line from the inside to the outside. Press your thumb in as shown. Whilst you are doing this, use the fingers of your left hand to rock the toes back and forth over your left thumb. For the left foot, swap hands and support with your right hand and work with your left.

Lung: sole (02)
For the right foot, support the top of the foot with your left hand and creep your right thumb along the area between the diaphragm line and shoulder line on the sole of the foot. Exchange hands for the left foot.

Lung: top of feet (03)
For the right foot, support the top of the foot with the fist of your left hand and creep your right index finger down the grooves on top of your foot. Swap hand positions for the left foot.

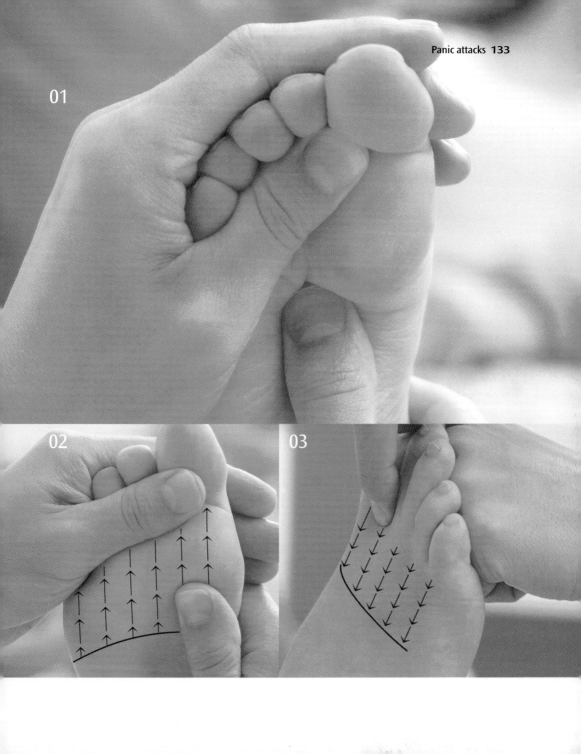

01

02

03

Period pains

Throughout the month the womb contracts and relaxes regularly. However, when your period is due the contractions become stronger in order to eliminate the lining of the womb. Menstruation becomes painful when the contractions are too strong or when there is an excess of the hormone-like substances called prostaglandins. Menstrual pains vary from a constant, dull lower backache to severe cramping in the lower abdominal area.

   You can control menstrual problems by changing certain eating habits, particularly in the week leading up to your period, and by taking plenty of exercise to increase blood circulation in the pelvic region.

REFLEXOLOGY

Uterus (01)
Work from the tip of the heel to the inside ankle bone with your index finger. The uterus reflex point is midway between heel and ankle bone.

Ovary (02)
Use your index finger to creep from the tip of the heel to the outside ankle bone. The actual reflex point for the ovary is halfway between the heel and ankle bone.

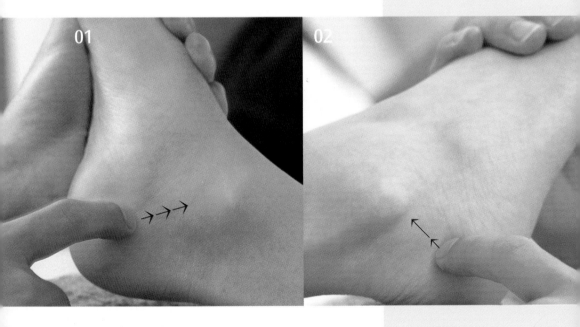

In general, eat a healthy, balanced diet (see pp.102–3) and take magnesium supplements to help relieve cramping as well as evening primrose oil, which contains linolenic acid, to combat PMS. The week before your period follow the eating guidelines on pp.46–7.

A reflexology foot treatment is excellent for relieving menstrual pain and will soon make you feel better, particularly if you are experiencing severe cramping. The most important reflexes to work are those relating to the reproductive system—the ovaries, fallopian tubes, and uterus—as well as the entire spine. To treat the hands and for general self-help see pp.46–7.

Fallopian tube *(03)*
Support the sole with your two thumbs and, pressing in with them, creep your third and index fingers of both hands across the top of the foot. Repeat three times.

Spine *(04)*
Creep up the inside edge of the foot as shown. Use the right thumb on the right foot and vice versa. Return to the big toe and creep your index finger up the outside edge.

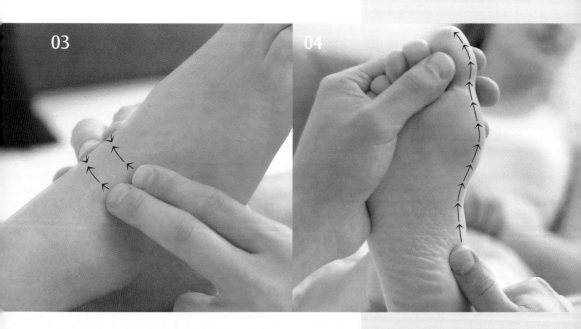

Throat infections

The tonsils, which are lymphatic glands, help prevent infection going further into the body. Pollution, cigarette fumes, and some food additives can irritate the lymphatic glands, so it is not unusual for the tonsils to become congested and swollen, thereby creating the perfect environment for bacteria and viruses to multiply. Swollen tonsils often lead to a very sore throat, headache (for treatment see pp.44–5 and pp.122–3), and fever, and overall make you feel extremely unwell. Tonsillitis can also develop into laryngitis or pharyngitis, resulting in "loss of voice". If this happens you must try not to speak, as it will make the condition worse and delay recovery.

Because the sinuses and throat are so closely linked, you must work both areas when treating any throat condition, either on the feet or on the hands. You should also treat the spine, particularly the cervical spine, to ease congestion and increase the blood supply to the throat.

GENERAL SELF-HELP
■ The most important things to do are to rest and drink plenty of pure spring water, particularly if you have laryngitis or pharyngitis.
■ If you have been diagnosed as having a streptococci throat infection, cook with plenty of garlic or take it as a supplement. Garlic has a strong antibacterial effect.
■ Goldenseal in capsule form is another herbal preparation offering natural antibiotic protection.
■ Remove mucus-forming foods from your diet and reduce your sugar intake to help your immune system.

ANTIBIOTICS
Only resort to antibiotic treatment if symptoms persist after you have tried reflexology for three or four days in combination with home remedies. As well as killing the bacteria causing the infection, antibiotics often upset the balance between certain "good" bacteria and fungi in the body. This can affect your digestive system and cause oral, intestinal, or vaginal thrush. Overuse of antibiotics also means that bacteria develop resistance, so stronger and stronger antibiotics have to be used to effectively fight off infection.

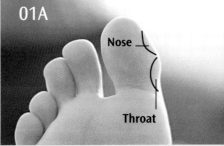

01A

Nose

Throat

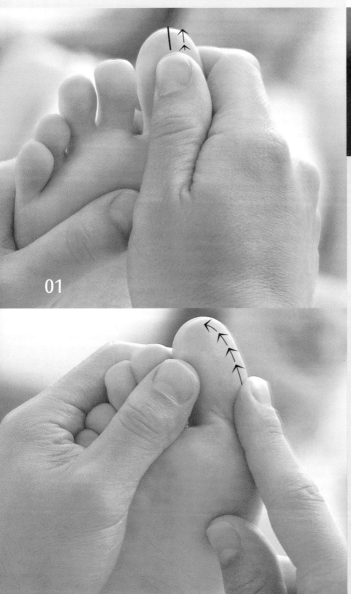

01

Sinuses & Throat *(01)*
Starting at the base of the big toe, creep up all the toes including the inside edge of the big toe to work the nose and throat (01A). When you reach the little toe, change hands and work back. For the right foot, hold the top of the foot with your left hand; for the left, swap hands.

Cervical spine *(02)*
The top seven vertebrae of the spine make up the cervical spine. To work this area, use your index finger to creep up the outside edge of the big toe in a fine movement. Repeat three or four times. On the right foot, support the top of the foot with your left hand and work with the right. For the left foot, change hands.

Useful addresses

To find out more about reflexology or to locate a professionally qualified reflexology practitioner, either nationally or internationally, contact:

Guild of Complementary Practitioners
Liddell House, Liddell Close,
Finchampstead, Berkshire
RG40 4NS, UK
Tel: +44 (0)118 973 5757
Fax: +44 (0)118 973 5767
Email: info@gepnet.com
Website: www.gepnet.com

If you have any questions or would like further information concerning reflexology books, charts, and videos, contact the author at:

Ann Gillanders Books
BSR (British School of Reflexology) Sales Ltd, 92 Sheering Road, Old Harlow, Essex CM17 0JW, UK
Tel: +44 (0)1279 429060
Fax: +44 (0)1279 445234
Email: ann@footreflexology.com
Website: www.footreflexology.com

If you are interested in finding out more about healthy eating, aromatherapy, homeopathy, naturopathy, or massage, contact the organizations below.

The Institute for Optimum Nutrition
Blades Court, Deodar Road,
London SW15 2NU, UK
Tel: +44 (0)20 8877 9993

The Aromatherapy Organisations Council
PO Box 19834, London SE25 6WF, UK
Tel: +44 (0)20 8251 7912

General Council and Register of Naturopaths
2 Goswell Road, Street,
Somerset BA16 0JG, UK
Tel: +44 (0)1458 840072

The Society of Homoeopaths
2 Artizan Road, Northampton
NN1 4HU, UK
Tel: +44 (0)1604 621400

British Massage Therapy Council
17 Rymers Lane, Oxford OX4 3JU, UK
Tel: +44 (0)1865 774123

Further reading

Batmanghelidj, Fereydoon,
Your Body's Many Cries for Water,
Tagman Press, 2000

Benson, Herbert,
The Relaxation Response,
Avon Books, 1976

Von Cramm, Dagmar,
Anti-Stress: Recipes for acid–alkaline balance, Gaia Books, 1999

Davies, Patricia,
Aromatherapy: An A to Z,
C. W. Daniel, 1998

Gillanders, Ann,
Compendium of Healing Points,
BSR Sales Ltd, 2001

Gillanders, Ann,
The Essential Guide to Foot and Hand Reflexology, BSR Sales Ltd, 1998

Gillanders, Ann,
Gateways to Health and Harmony,
BSR Sales Ltd, 1997

Gillanders, Ann,
Reflexology: A step-by-step guide,
Gaia Books, 1995

Ingham, Christine,
Panic Attacks,
Thorsons, 1993

Kirsta, Alix,
The Book of Stress Survival,
Gaia Books, 1986

Lavery, Sheila,
The Healing Power of Sleep,
Gaia Books, 1997

Lidell, Lucy,
The New Book of Massage,
Ebury Press, 2000

Mabey, Richard,
New Age Herbalist,
Simon & Schuster, 2001

Mojay, Gabriel,
Aromatherapy for Healing the Spirit,
Gaia Books, 1999

Nice, Jill,
Herbal Remedies & Home Comforts,
Piatkus, 1990

Wells, Judith,
The Food Bible,
Quadrille Publishing, 1998

Index

Acknowledgements

Author's acknowledgements
My thanks to David for advising the team during the photo shoot. I would also like to thank Susanna Abbott for the professional and sensitive approach in editing this book and Phil Gamble for his superb artistic design.

Publisher's acknowledgements
Gaia Books would like to thank Lynn Bresler for proofreading and indexing; Läyne Kuirk-Schwarz-Waad and Hannah Santos Lã at Planet Organic, Torrington Street, London; Steven Zarka; the models Ashley Khoo, Susan Alston, and Suzi Langhorne.